TOUGH DECISIONS

TOUGH DECISIONS *A Casebook*

in Medical Ethics

JOHN M. FREEMAN
KEVIN McDONNELL

New York   Oxford
OXFORD UNIVERSITY PRESS
1987

Oxford University Press

Oxford New York Toronto
Delhi Bombay Calcutta Madras Karachi
Petaling Jaya Singapore Hong Kong Tokyo
Nairobi Dar es Salaam Cape Town
Melbourne Auckland

and associated companies in
Beirut Berlin Ibadan Nicosia

Library of Congress Cataloging-in-Publication Data
Freeman, John Mark.
Tough decisions.
1. Medical ethics—Case studies. 2. Medicine,
Clinical—Decision making—Case studies. 3. Decision
making (Ethics)—Case studies. I. McDonnell, Kevin.
II. Title. [DNLM: 1. Decision Making. 2. Ethics,
Medical. W 50 F855t]
R725.5.F74 1987 174'.2 86-31190
ISBN 0-19-504255-7
ISBN 0-19-504256-5 (pbk.)

9 8 7 6 5 4 3 2 1

Printed in the United States of America
on acid-free paper

We dedicate this book to the many children and their parents who, as we have struggled together through difficult times and tough decisions, have taught us to be better, wiser, and more humble decision makers.

We further dedicate this book to our wives, Elaine and Carol, and our children for their forbearance while we have learned, taught, and written.

Preface

This book is the fruit of a dialogue between a philosopher and a physician, a theorist and a practitioner, about the practice and teaching of medical ethics. The traditional teaching of ethics starts by laying a foundation in ethical theory and then applies one or more of these theories to fully presented cases. This approach seemed to us too abstract, with the theories being simply laid over the cases. An alternative approach often begins with cases, each one illustrative of a single moral theory or medical-ethical situation. We found these presentations of cases similar to the cases in an appellate court, lacking the drama, subtlety, and conflict of the original courtroom, and too brief to provide a sufficient sense of the interconnections between moral, medical, and social problems.

There seemed no better solution than to write our own book. The cases in this book force the reader to look ahead, rather than to look back over a completed story. Our case presentations are modeled on the adventure books and computer games that ask the reader to take part in the story. We place the reader in the middle of a complex problem. The reader's decisions change the course of the story in much the same way as decisions about medical care can change the course of life and death. We ask the reader to face both medical and moral uncertainty. Medicine is an art as well as a science, and the outcome of medical decisions is not entirely predictable. The morality of decisions made must be compatible with the uncertainty of outcome.

Instead of attempting to deduce solutions from abstract principles, we have taken a more empirical and inductive approach. Medical care is tailored to the needs of a given patient here and now. While general principles of diagnosis and therapy are always involved, medicine never loses touch with the individual patient. In this casebook, therefore, while remaining well aware that decisions are related to principles, we have maintained a focus on the moral decision maker.

We have tried to keep principles in closer relation to the cases by putting relevant philosophical views into the mouths of characters in the story. We tell each story from the point of view of a single character and invite the reader to assume that perspective. Other characters advocate ethical theories or courses of action with appropriate justification. We use an editorial voice only when we could find no other way to develop an option or point of view.

The number of cases in this book is limited. This makes it possible to describe the medical situation in lay terms and to explain at least in part the social and family background for each case. Another advantage of treating a small number of cases in detail is that it forces the reader to see that a case may present not one, but a number of moral dilemmas, and that the resolution of one dilemma may create another. The reader is also forced to see the interconnections between moral problems and moral theories. The book's Contents shows which of the major issues of medical ethics are covered in each case, but we have tried to keep the issues in their native, intertwined state rather than in abstract isolation from each other.

Our cases are amalgams of actual events sufficiently disguised to preserve confidentiality. They are condensations that present various options. In any real situation, there are multiple choices and myriad gradations of each choice. For the purposes of this book we have limited options and outcomes to representative examples. Some of the proposed choices may be illegal or suggest departures from standard medicine. Just as in real life, one must take these possibilities into account. Finally, we ask readers not to confuse the views of the characters or the prepared solutions with the views of the authors.

Chapter 14 discusses some of the major approaches to moral theory and suggests further reading in medical ethics. In Chapter 15 we argue that since the outcome cannot be known at the time of making the decision, the virtue of the decision lies in the process by which it is made. We hope readers will use these chapters in dealing with the difficult questions posed by the cases.

<table>
<tr><td>*Baltimore, Md.*</td><td>J.M.F.</td></tr>
<tr><td>*Notre Dame, Ind.*</td><td>K.McD.</td></tr>
<tr><td>*November 1986*</td><td></td></tr>
</table>

Acknowledgments

To Mrs. Mary E. Edwards, John Freeman's administrative secretary, who has revised the many drafts of this book without complaint, we offer our special thanks and appreciation.

We thank Professor Charles Kay, his students, and Kevin McDonnell's students who have used the cases and offered many excellent suggestions.

We are also grateful to friends and colleagues—among them Professors Ruth Faden, Peg Falls, Elizabeth Linehan, Joseph Lombardi, Stuart Warner, and Morton Winston—who reviewed chapters and offered encouragement and helpful criticism.

Jeffrey House and the editors at Oxford University Press have been persistently and cordially helpful.

The faults that remain, of course, we acknowledge as our own.

ACKNOWLEDGMENTS

Contents

Contents

Contents

"letting die" just a slow way of killing? May a respirator be removed? May nasogastric feeding be discontinued? Is euthanasia acceptable?

Contents

Introduction

This book is about the difficult moral decisions that arise ever more frequently in the course of medical practice. The dilemmas we depict in this book are not the only moral issues in medicine and are probably not even the most common, but they are among the most dramatic. Although we have presented them as fictional cases in order to explore their many nuances, they are all based on first-hand experience. They represent amalgams of true cases we have seen, discussed in depth, and often personally managed. Some are like the dramatic cases played out in the newspaper or on nightly television, but in this book we do not merely allow the reader to look on while others decide. We cast the reader in the role of decision maker. What happens depends on your decisions.

The book's format is intended to give readers a clear sense of the pressures that come to bear on clinical decision making. The cases are interrupted at critical points, and the reader is asked to make a decision. The reader's choice directs him or her to one of several paths through the case. Thus, as in real life, he or she determines the course of events and sometimes the outcome. We assume that the reader wants to do the right thing but faces the problem of determining what that is. The dialogue of the cases embodies various perspectives grounded in various moral theories, offering different views of what is right in given medical situations.

For physicians, deciding what to do in such situations was once easier. One followed the Hippocratic oath.

> I will follow that regimen which, according to my ability and judgement, I consider for the benefit of my patients, and abstain from whatever is deleterious and mischievous.
>
> Oath of Hippocrates
> Translated by Sir Francis Adams

When the oath was written, there were few effective remedies available to physicians. So long as they refrained from intentionally doing harm or intentionally doing more harm than good, physicians could be said to practice "good medicine." Medical science and technology, however, have enabled physicians to prolong life or cure disease for many patients who were formerly beyond help. We now find ourselves asking whether there are situations in which the use of life-prolonging therapies may not be beneficial and may even be harmful.

Nonetheless, it remains a basic tenet of medicine that the physician must always care for his or her patients. "To care" is defined in Webster's Dictionary as "to be concerned about," and that concern should never be terminated. But the term "to care" is often misused in medical parlance as a contraction for "to provide care," that is, to intervene or to do something active—for instance, to start a respirator, to use medications, or to begin tube feeding. There is an important distinction between the care and concern that should always be provided and the technical intervention, which may not benefit the patient.

Having stated the obvious—that physicians must always care for their patients and do what is to their benefit—how do we define "benefit?" Beyond the minimum care required to sustain the dignity of a human being, the meaning of "benefit" depends on the facts of the individual case and the interpretation and understanding of those facts by physicians, patients, families, and society.

Physicians are routinely involved in decisions about appropriate care. The question may be one of starting, continuing, or withdrawing therapy. Some physicians want to base their decisions on *what* will happen, that is, on the outcome. Others want to designate a particular person—for example, the patient, the parent or family, or the courts—*who* will make the decision. Our thesis, however, is that *how* the decision is made is most important. It is the process of decision making that counts.

Whatever the decision is, whoever makes it, and on whatever basis it is made, it must be a moral decision. How does one assure that the decision will be moral? How does one review decisions already made to assess whether they are moral?

We start with the assumption that most of us are basically decent people. But often individuals are unwittingly insensitive or unaware of the issues that should guide decisions. Ethical theory provides guidelines for moral decision making, but to use these guidelines, the decision maker must have some grounding in ethics. He or she must have some awareness of the arguments and theories that form the boundaries of what is moral.

Two factors have heightened the problematic character of the decisions we now face in medicine. The first is the development and widespread availability of new technology. It is now possible to transplant hearts and kidneys, to maintain breathing and heartbeat with a respirator, and to save one-pound babies. In the past twenty years these therapies have moved from speculative gleams in the eyes of a few researchers to well-established and widely available therapies.

As our ability to perform these "medical miracles" improves, we must increasingly face moral decisions about the development of this technology and its legitimate use. Should we put a virtually brain-dead patient on the respirator? Should we try one more therapy for a patient's cancer? Should we operate on a newborn child with many severe problems? Are such procedures a benefit to the patient, or do they merely prolong his or her misery? These are not technical questions but human and moral ones of the highest order.

Hand in hand with advances in technology have come changes in social attitudes toward medicine and the practice of medicine. Very few people are fortunate enough to have family physicians who have known and cared for them over long periods of time, physicians whose attitudes and values they know and share. The great mobility of our population and the fact that more and more conditions are treated by specialists have made it less likely that health care providers will know the attitudes and the moral and cultural diversity of their patients and the effects of these on medical decision making. In addition, patients and their families want to be more fully informed and to participate more actively in their health care decisions.

Many difficult medical decisions arise, therefore, from the increasing ambiguity that technology has introduced, multiplied by increasing public and private conflicts over which courses of action are morally appropriate. How should we determine what to do? If two people decide differently, is one of them wrong? Can good, reasonable people confronting the same dilemma reach different conclusions and make different decisions?

Moral philosophy attempts to develop organized ways of resolving these questions by using the theories of Aristotle, Kant, the utilitarians, and others. Ethicists, philosophers, and theologians are the students and interpreters of these varied approaches, many working to develop and apply new guidelines for modern problems.

But increasingly faced with different moral decisions, health care professionals often ask too much of ethicists. They ask for specific answers to specific problems. And they ask not just the standard questions like, "Should I treat this newborn infant?," "Should I turn off Mr. X's respirator?," or "Should I try this new drug for Mrs. Y's cancer?," but also more subtle questions like, "How should I bias the information to parents so they make the appropriate decision?" and "What are my responsibilities when the family or relatives are making what I believe is the wrong decision?" Ethics does not answer specific questions like these. Ethical theory is not designed to tell us what to do in a given situation. Rather, it provides a framework for making decisions. It delineates the boundaries of morally acceptable behavior and the guidelines under which decisions should be made. We believe that ethical theory is meant to tell us *how* to make a decision and what the ingredients and bases of a morally acceptable decision are, not what decision to make.

It is the lack of understanding of what ethics is intended to do that often leads health care professionals to be impatient with the lack of answers from ethicists. But this is not the ethicist's problem. The ethicist was asked the wrong question. Health care professionals should not be asking what to do; they should be asking the ethicist to clarify the bases for deciding what to do.

Even without knowing or appealing directly to ethical theory, however, health care professionals must justify their decisions in some terms—in terms of rights, duties, benefits, or some other staple of moral philosophy. Even when we appeal to our feelings and intuition, even when we invoke the Hippocratic oath and review our professional obligations, we are utilizing, implicitly, philosophical concepts and concerns about what should be done. There is no method of explaining or justifying a decision without using some of the elements and language of ethical theory.

A further reason for the health care professional's frequent impatience with ethics is the pressure of time on the physician's decision-making progress. In many situations a decision must be made without full information about many elements that may be morally important in the process. An inability to decide or a delay engendered by a prolonged search for missing elements may constitute a decision by default. During the delay the patient may die, or the opportunity for intervention may pass.

To simulate situations occurring in modern medicine, we have tried to add the pressure of time to our cases. As in real life, we have placed the reader in the middle of complex problems, in messy family situations, in the context of a conflicted society. We have shown how medical decisions are confounded by the uncertainty of outcome, whatever decision is made. The book's format is designed to allow the reader's decisions to change the course of the case in much the same way as medical decisions can change the course of life and death. Since the outcome of medical decisions is not entirely predictable, we ask the reader to face both medical and moral uncertainty. Morality is also a practical study, concerned with the impact of the decisions we make on our own and others' lives.

We hope that students, by going through these exercises conscientiously, pausing to think through and justify the forced decisions, will become more sympathetic and empathetic to all participants in the decision-making process and more sensitive to the moral dilemmas they face.

Introduction

Through practice we believe that a person can become a better decision maker, aware of the possibility that others with the same information may come to different conclusions. One then has to develop tolerance to alternative decisions, but in doing so must also define the limits of one's own tolerance within the range of possible decisions, and in this way decide which are morally acceptable and which are not.

In defending their decision, readers will have to use the language of rights, obligations, and benefits—words that have roots in the language of philosophy and ethics. We hope that this will lead many to a desire to know and understand these ethical traditions.

To paraphrase Kant, "Experience without theory is blind. Theory without experience is empty." In this book we have tried to provide readers with both experience (albeit simulated) and some theory, with the opportunity to think about problems, to face them in realistic situations, and then to think about them again with others who can bring scrutiny to bear on the quality of thought.

A Note to the Reader

We want you to experience some of the uncertainty and tension that surround genuine medical decisions. To this end, we ask that you follow the instructions given in each case. After reading some narrative material, you will reach a decision point. Think very carefully at this point, and then commit yourself to one of the courses of action proposed. (The cases are set up so that not deciding is clearly as much a decision as any other.) Then follow the implications of your decision by turning to the section indicated.

This book is not meant to be read continuously from beginning to end. Reading straight through would frustrate the whole purpose of the case presentations, which is to place you in the position of a decision maker. At the decision points you should pause to ask: Are you doing the right thing? How would you justify the decision you are making? Is your decision consistent with decisions you have made in other cases? In your own life? Is it appropriate to your role in the case? Have you weighed the revelant factors properly?

TOUGH DECISIONS

Chapter 1

Maggie

Margaret O'Sullivan, known as Maggie, was as lively as one could be at age 74. As a resident in the family practice program, you meet her at the retirement home on your rounds with her private physician, Dr. Loeb. Dr. Loeb visits all his patients every month and checks each week for minor illnesses or to adjust medications. You stop by every day to monitor things and to learn about the problems of elderly patients.

You especially enjoy Maggie because she is not a complainer. How could she be? As a dedicated fan of the Chicago Cubs, she knows the meaning of hope in the face of adversity. She can usually be found holding court in "her" corner of the residents' lounge. Maggie is on medication to control a slightly erratic heartbeat, and you find yourself, quite unnecessarily, stopping in the lounge to ask how she is doing. She is always "Just fine, thank you." Sometimes, in addition to the latest word on the Cubbies, she will add that she is lucky to be better off than poor Mr. So and So who was just trucked off to the hospital. Maggie is a good deal more realistic about medicine than about baseball.

"No one will ever see him again," she will mutter, "though it'll be a long time before he's dead. You doctors and your infernal machines. Thinking about it is enough to make a body sick. But you know what I want. I've told you, and I've told Doctor Loeb. I don't mind taking a few pills now and again, but I do mind nurses and doctors running around and pounding on an old lady's chest, and all those damn machines. I don't want any of that resuscitation stuff. When it's my time, I just want to go. My time will come when the Cubbies win another pennant. And since that may take a little while, I have to keep in shape. The best way to do that, you know, is to keep away from you doctors."

"You know," she said another time, "my nephew is a lawyer, and I've been talking to him about all this resuscitation and machine stuff. I saw about the living will in the paper. He says the legislature hasn't passed it in this state. But I told him what I thought and how I wanted to go. He said I could send him a letter with all that in it, so I told him to write the letter and I'd sign it. Well, he did. I also changed my will. I put it in there that, if I were resuscitated and kept going, my estate should sue the doctors so they would pay for my care while I was on those machines. It's terrible to be hooked up to the damn things, but then to have to pay for it is just too much. I also told Brian, my nephew, that he should try to sue any doctor who did any of that stuff to me. Brian said he would and, you know, Brian is a very good lawyer. I'm not saying any of this to threaten you or anything, I'm just telling you how I feel. I think it's pretty clear how I feel."

It certainly is clear. And as she tells the stories of her friends in the home and how they died, it becomes even clearer that her views are well founded. In light of what Maggie has been saying all along, what happened to her shows the gods' sense of irony.

When you went through the home with Dr. Loeb yesterday, Maggie had left word that she wanted to see him. "My ticker isn't right," she said, "and would he please stop by and take a listen."

Dr. Loeb found Maggie in her room, which was unusual. She was sitting in a lounge chair by the window reading *The Sporting News*. She said that she thought her heart had been skipping beats and that it was running too fast. He took her pulse, which was 100, and listened to her heart. There did, indeed, seem to be an arrhythmia.

"Sounds like you need different pills, Maggie," he said. "We'll change the medicine. That ought to take care of it. We don't need any tests right now, except an electrocardiogram (EKG). I know how you just love those machines. I'll have my young friend here fuss a bit with your meds, and everything will be OK."

Out in the hall, Dr. Loeb said, "I'm sure it's nothing much. Don't get her all upset with a lot of tests and stuff. Move her down to the infirmary and work through some of the usual medications and see if you can straighten it out. It doesn't sound bad, and you are here every day to keep an eye on things. See you next week."

You had heard the same arrythmias as Dr. Loeb and were pretty confident you could handle things. You stopped back in to tell Maggie that she would be just fine, and that you'd start her on a new drug in the morning.

The same afternoon you consulted one of the cardiologists at the hospital who suggested that you look at some of the newer drugs for arrhythmia. She mentioned two she had found very effective and thought you should read up on them. That night you read over the literature on both drugs and thought one looked promising for Maggie's problem. It called for beginning treatment with a single injection that would establish a load of the drug in the bloodstream. Afterward, blood levels could be maintained with two to four pills per day.

You felt that the drug would make Maggie feel better quickly. It would be good for Maggie's morale. She didn't like to feel sickly.

First thing this morning, you called the pharmacy and ordered the drug delivered to the home's infirmary. You also called the nurse's station at the infirmary and left a message with the clerk that you would come in later to start Maggie on a new medication. Around 10 A.M. you tell Maggie about the new medication. While you are sitting in the nurse's station writing the new order, the nurse takes the medicine down the hall to give Maggie an injection.

The home's infirmary is peaceful and quiet, a welcome relief from the pace at the hospital. You are just getting up to leave when a nurse comes flying out of Maggie's room. "Call a code on Maggie," she shouts to the nurse's station. You rush into Maggie's room to find her slumped over in bed, the sports pages still clutched in her hand. She has passed out. Her heart sounds are wildly arrythmic and her respiration extremely shallow. Her skin is cold and clammy and has lost all its color. Maggie is having a severe reaction to the medication. She is in shock.

In practically no other situation could you conceive of ordering resuscitation for Maggie. Had no one witnessed her fibrillation, the chances of a good recovery would be very small. These were the kinds of cases Maggie had talked about. However, when there was an immediate report and a physician on the scene, the chances of a good outcome were much improved. You had handled several such situations, but it is not clear how well the staff of the home is trained.

Another point in favor of resuscitation is that the cause of Maggie's problem is clear. You had just reviewed all the literature on the drug and knew that its action could be reversed. In the meantime, standard resuscitation procedures could be followed.

A final point in favor of resuscitation is your liability and that of the home for Maggie's death. Since you had ordered the drug, you would be liable. Since you were working under Dr. Loeb's supervision, he would be liable. And, of course, the nurse and the retirement home might be liable as well. Maggie's nephew Brian is, you had heard, one of the smartest lawyers in town. He might just find it a good idea to increase the value of Maggie's estate regardless of her instructions not to resuscitate.

You really do not like to think about this last point, preferring to concentrate on what Maggie wanted. But her desires suddenly became very ambiguous. She would have a very good chance, at least 75 percent, of coming out of this thing with minimal, if any, damage. She would have perhaps a 10-percent chance of ending up with a prolonged unconsciousness ending in death. The 15 percent left over would be moderate damage—a substantially weakened heart and a damaged brain. She would be weak, feeble, and confused, but she would be conscious of her condition and have some sense of how she arrived there. This last state would be the worst of all, the one Maggie feared.

It was September 1, 1984, and the Chicago Cubs were leading their division by four and a half games.

* * *

What should you do? Should you resuscitate Maggie?

Remember, she clearly told you she did *not* want to be resuscitated. She did not want "those damn machines." But is this the situation she had in mind? This is an allergic reaction, one that you can easily treat. Her chances of complete recovery are good. The chances if you don't treat are terrible—for her, and maybe for you.

If you decide to resuscitate Maggie, are you making this decision: (1) Because if she had known about this situation she would have wanted to be resuscitated? (2) Because in this situation the only reasonable decision would be to want to be resuscitated? Therefore, you act on her behalf paternalistically. Or (3) because her predicament is your fault and you need to protect yourself and everyone else?

If you decide to resuscitate Maggie, turn to the section entitled "You Decide on a Full-Scale Resuscitation" (p. 9).

Why would you decide *not* to resuscitate Maggie? Is her refusal absolute? Have you extended it to a situation she could not possibly have anticipated? Would following Maggie's clear wishes not to be resuscitated be an adequate moral defense? If you decide *not* to resuscitate Maggie, read the next section.

You Decide Not to Resuscitate

You walk out to the hall swearing under your breath. You decide, however, that Maggie's wishes were very clear and should be honored. You walk quickly to the nurse's desk and tell the charge nurse to cancel the code. She protests.

"You can't do that. We're responsible. You can't just walk out on this thing and leave us hanging. Maggie had an unusual reaction to the medication. We could reverse it, resuscitate Maggie, and there's a good chance she will be OK. We've got to follow through on the code. We can ask questions afterward."

Although you hate to do it, the only way to settle the thing is to pull rank. "I'm the doctor," you say, "and I'll take the responsibility. Maggie did not want to re resuscitated—she was always clear about that. She is a no-code patient and that's it—no code."

"Well," says the nurse, "then you tell the family. What are you going to say when they ask how Aunt Maggie died? Are you going to tell them she had a bad reaction to the medication? We're certainly going to make sure that the nursing notes show that you canceled the resuscitation, and that you were responsible for the change in Maggie's meds. Maggie's death is your fault."

* * *

What *are* you going to tell the family? Are you going to tell the whole story? Are you thinking that the family will respect you for telling the truth right at the start and recognize that you were doing your best to follow Maggie's wishes? Or are you going to spare the family the details, telling them that Maggie's heart "just gave out," and filling them in on your attempt to adjust the medication and your decision not to resuscitate only so far as they press you for details? After all, there is nothing more to be done for Maggie. Your career would be a lot smoother without a malpractice settlement during your residency. Susan, the new nurse, the nursing home, and even Dr. Loeb would be happier not to have to face all the hassle and guilt of malpractice proceedings. And it is not as though the family needed the money.

What obligation do you have to tell the truth? How strong is your obligation in this case when telling the truth will probably only hurt people? Does Maggie's family have a right to the truth? Where does that right come from? Think about the moral issues involved before making your decision.

If you decide to tell the whole truth, see the section entitled "Heads" (p. 8).

If you decide to edit the truth and not reveal the full facts, flip a coin. If it comes up heads, go to the "Heads" section (p. 8). If it comes up tails, read the following section.

Tails

Tails—you win! The family does not press too hard. Only Brian, Maggie's nephew, pushes a little. But when you talk to him about the difficult decision you faced and how you decided to respect Maggie's wishes, he compliments you on the decision.

"Every profession has its tough calls," he says. "People on the outside don't really understand how it is. You just have to put your faith in those who know."

About a month later, Brian phones you. He tells you that Maggie's will left $250,000 to the home. There is also a discretionary fund, and he would like you to have $2000. The home is having a little ceremony to accept the bequest and to honor Maggie. The family and the administration and staff of the home will all be there. Brian asks you to please write up a little talk about Maggie and how she died.

It is the seventh of October, 1984, and the Chicago Cubs have just lost the National League playoffs to the San Diego Padres.

* * *

Reflect on your decisions in this case. Are you comfortable with them? Were they good decisions, or just expedient? What was the moral basis for your decisions? Can moral theory ever justify lying or telling only part of the truth?

Heads

It is now a month since you decided not to resuscitate Maggie O'Sullivan. The lawyers call their procedure "discovery"; more lurid but accurate medical terms come to mind. You are seated in the home's conference room with the home's lawyer on one side and a lawyer from the university (since you are a member of its residency program) on the other. Both have made it clear in conversation beforehand that they think you made a dreadful mistake and that the best thing they can hope for is to limit the damage. They have very different ideas, of course, as to whose damage should be limited. Maggie's nephew Brian was there as well. He was pressing the suit, and an attorney from his firm was conducting the session.

Dr. Loeb completes his testimony, in which he says that the decision not to resuscitate Maggie was a tragic mistake, if not criminally negligent. He grants that Maggie made a request not to be resuscitated, but points out that it is a doctor's responsibility to put that request in context. In the context in which Maggie died, he states, there was close to a 100-percent chance of survival and an excellent chance of happy survival. When Maggie's view of resuscitation is read in this context, Dr. Loeb finds it "hard, even impossible, to conceive how someone could not have called for a full-scale resuscitation effort. Maggie's Chicago Cubs didn't quit; I'm sure Maggie would have wanted to carry on."

The charge nurse is next to appear. She points out that they pleaded with you to resuscitate Maggie. They insisted that the home had all the required equipment and trained personnel to handle such situations. They also said that, having researched the literature on the drug you ordered, its action was reversible with the use of other medications that were available in the home's infirmary. They insisted that they were ready to begin a full-scale effort to resuscitate Maggie when you stopped them. They had tried, of course, to phone Dr. Loeb immediately, but they could not reach him until it was clearly too late.

You are now sworn in to give testimony. Think about your testimony as you might give it, responding to the obvious questions and putting your decision in the best possible light. Be sure to include the moral justification for your medical decisions.

* * *

You might like to see the outcome if you had decided to resuscitate Maggie. If so, read the next section.

You Decide on a Full-Scale Resuscitation

You act immediately and decisively. You order the nurse to crank Maggie's bed down and you begin external chest compression. The nurse brings the red "crash" cart with the defibrillator. As you are putting the paddles on Maggie's chest, the head nurse decides to give you grief about resuscitating.

"You know," she says, "that Maggie is a no code. She does not want to be resuscitated. I know that Dr. Loeb has been over that with her and that Maggie signed a statement in her chart. No matter how she got into trouble, there is no justification for trying to resuscitate her. Her wishes are clear, and we should honor them. I don't see how I can mobilize the resuscitation team until you convince me that this is the right thing to do."

Just what you need at a resuscitation effort, you think to yourself, a running philosophical commentary on the right of patients to refuse heroic medical therapy. What you say to her, however, is quite unphilosophical. "I'm the doctor, and I'm in charge. I want a full resuscitation effort, and I want it stat—now."

It takes several electric shocks to get Maggie's heart beat stabilized;

the process takes so long that you fear things are not going to go well for her. You are right.

Three days later you go on hospital rounds with Dr. Loeb. Maggie had been transferred to the hospital, and Dr. Loeb wanted you to see how things turned out. As luck would have it Brian, Maggie's nephew, has stopped by on his way to the office. Maggie seems to have shrunk to half her previous size. She is so pale and wrinkled that she almost disappears into the bed linens. Her voice is weak, and she is not very lucid. She manages to mumble things like "Why am I here? Where am I? What are you doing to me?" All of this is mixed with assorted groans and incoherent mumblings.

Brian is hostile from the start. He begins by confronting Dr. Loeb. "Perhaps we can talk out in the hall, where we won't disturb Aunt Maggie," he says when you and Dr. Loeb finish your examination. Dr. Loeb nods, flips through the chart, reading carefully the cardiologist's report on the EKG, and reaches down to squeeze Maggie's hand. Then the three of you adjourn to the corridor.

"Aunt Maggie always made it clear to me, and I am certain she made it crystal clear to you, that the state she is in now is something that she would abhor. She was very explicit about it in the past and, so far as I can see, she still feels the same way. Although she is not completely coherent now, she does seem to have some idea of what happened. She is very distressed and upset. In the 15 minutes before you came in, she was whining and mumbling that 'It's awful,' and 'I hate being this way.' I intend to find out how all this happened. I want to know why you acted as you did—why you resuscitated her against her explicit instructions and the written orders that she not be resuscitated. Furthermore, following her directions, I intend to pursue the matter of who is to pay for her care. You know that she thought it unconscionable for you doctors to keep people alive like this against their will. I am on my way to the office now to consult with some of my colleagues about bringing a civil action against the two of you and the home for all of Aunt Maggie's expenses for the rest of her life."

Dr. Loeb winces at this last remark. Instead of being hostile, however, he just seems sad. He attempts to calm Brian.

"These things are just unpredictable, Brian. I can understand how angry you are, but there is nothing to be done now. It was a judgment call and, under the circumstances, it seems to me that my young colleague was correct. I would have done the same thing myself. There was a nurse with Maggie when her heart went into fibrillation and a doctor was coming down the corridor. There was a very good chance things would have worked out better than this, that Maggie would have been just fine, but you can never be sure. We have done the best we could. Maggie is not on any machines, and we don't intend to put her on any. She is not in great shape mentally or emotionally; I'm sure she has sustained some brain damage but, at this point we can't tell how much. She certainly won't be the same as she used to be, but at least she is still alive. She is still with us, and she is not in any pain.

"I know this isn't what any of us wanted, but we don't always get what we want. I know you want to take it out on us now, but maybe you'll calm down and see that nothing can change the situation Maggie is in."

Brian is not much mollified. "Patients have rights, you know. And from a legal point of view, their primary right is to refuse treatment they don't want. I am going to work vigorously to see that Aunt Maggie's rights and wishes are respected and that she not be forced to pay for the abuse of her rights. I'll be seeing both of you again."

As Dr. Loeb watches Brian stride down the corridor, he said softly, "Most of them calm down sooner or later."

"I think you did the right thing, or at least the only thing you could do. Under the circumstances you couldn't just stand there and watch her die. You did have a good shot at it."

* * *

Was your decision to resuscitate Maggie a good decision? It might have had a different result. She might have been just fine, or she might have died anyway; as sometimes happens, she did neither. Do any of these outcomes make the decision good or bad?

Does the moral quality of your decision depend on the outcome? Rethink your previous decisions. Are you still comfortable and confident about your decisions considering Maggie's current state? Do you want another chance to make a different decision? If so, go back to page 6 and try again. If not, outline how you will explain and justify your decision in response to Brian's outrage.

If you are satisfied with your decision and its moral basis, turn to the long-term outcome. Flip a coin to see what that outcome will be. If the coin comes up heads, read the next section, entitled "Heads." If it comes up tails, turn to the section entitled "Tails" (p. 12).

Heads

Three months have passed, and Maggie is back at the nursing home. There were a few rocky days when Maggie was confused and at times combative, but she gradually came around. Within a week she is back almost to her old self; within two weeks she returns to the retirement home.

The Cubs, she learns, lost and "as I told you, Doctor, I'm going to be around till they win the pennant. By the way," she says for the fourth time, "if I haven't already told you, I'm awfully glad you were here when I needed you. You're such a good doctor. Brian is still all upset about everything that went on, but he'll calm down. See you tomorrow."

* * *

If you are curious about what would have happened if you had decided *not* to resuscitate Maggie, return to the section "You Decide Not to Resuscitate" (p. 6) and start again.

Tails

Three months have passed since the problems with Maggie began, and she is still in the hospital. Maggie has come around a bit, but remains confused and rambling. Since she can no longer walk, she's confined to bed or a wheelchair. This has been one of the factors in the two episodes of pneumonia that have set back her recovery. She remembers her friends at the retirement home and keeps asking to "go back home," but the hospital staff just hasn't been able to get her well enough. It's getting harder to visit her every week. How do you respond when all she asks is "Why, Doctor? Why?"

* * *

If you are unhappy with the outcome and think it might have been better *not* to have resuscitated Maggie, return to the section "You Decide Not to Resuscitate" (p. 6) and try again.

Chapter 2

Monica

"I spent most of yesterday at the National Library of Medicine reading the 120 most recent articles on medulloblastoma in this age group. I've talked to the head of pediatric neuro-oncology at the Farber Center in Boston and to people in Philadelphia, San Francisco, Johns Hopkins, and M.D. Anderson. I also had a long conversation with one of my friends on the staff at the Cancer Institute. It's not at all clear to me that you can give Monica much of a chance at a decent life. There's only a 20-percent chance of her surviving, and 50 percent of those survivors are retarded and brain damaged. I don't think you should operate!"

Dr. Peters was going to be a great trial to you. Brilliant, driven, aggressive—he had put all of these attributes in high gear and learned all there was to know about medulloblastoma in the two days since you had admitted his 2-year-old daughter with the presumptive diagnosis.

Monica, a beautiful 2-year-old brunette, was admitted late Friday evening after a two-week history of unsteady gait that had gradually gotten worse. She became sleepy and began vomiting. The pediatrician at first thought it was a virus but, on examining her eyes, evidence of increased intracranial pressure was found, and she was immediately referred to Metropolitan General. A brain scan Saturday morning revealed what looked like a large tumor in the back of her head, probably one of the most malignant types—a medulloblastoma. An operation was scheduled for the next morning to confirm the suspected diagnosis and to remove the bulk of the tumor before irradiation. A tumor of that type and in that location cannot be completely removed.

"Just a minute, Dr. Peters," you say, "what do you mean we shouldn't operate tomorrow? You mean we should just stand here and let Monica die? I'm upset enough that it's taken so long to get her on the operating room schedule. If you hadn't insisted on the chairman's operating she would have been out of the recovery room already. We've had to watch her like a hawk; there's not much room between life and death with a tumor that size back there."

"Listen," said Peters, "I'm not in a good mood, and I don't have much patience with residents just now. I don't have to justify myself to you or your interns. Dr. Longsworth is in charge and I'll deal with him. You just take good care of Monica until Dr. Longsworth and I decide what's best."

It's Sunday morning, but you ask the head nurse and the hospital chaplain to join you on rounds to discuss Monica's case. Dr. Peters is getting on everyone's nerves.

"Reverend," you begin, "we have a problem on the ward and we need your help. Monica Peters is a cute 2-year-old admitted two days ago with a brain tumor. She's scheduled for an operation tomorrow and her father, who is an obstetrical resident at Eastern, now says he doesn't want the operation—he wants to let her die. All of us are very upset about this. Monica is a beautiful little girl. We can't let her die without doing anything. What do we do now?"

Reverend Carlisle is a rotund, friendly, pipe-smoking, former Unitarian pastor who has been the hospital chaplain for the past 10 years. A good friend of the students, nurses, and residents, he has become the unofficial confessor to many.

"Well," he mumbles through the haze of his pipe smoke, "that's a tough one. Good decisions depend on good facts. Why doesn't Dr. Peters want the operation for his daughter?"

"The facts are pretty much as Dr. Peters himself stated," you reply. "I haven't been able to do all the reading and consulting he's done, but if this is a medulloblastoma, the literature shows only a 20-percent, 5-year survival in children this age. This is based on removing as much of the tumor as possible and giving radiation to the whole brain and spinal cord. The problem is that giving radiation to the young brain has a substantial chance of causing retardation and even strokes, so only 50 percent of the survivors are normal. That's why a year ago we started a new policy of not giving radiation to children this age, but only chemotherapy. It's too early to know the long-term results of this change. The number of children who survive with chemotherapy may not be as great as with radiation, but deferring radiation until age 3 or 4 should improve the quality of life of the survivors."

"You said, 'if this is a medulloblastoma.' Don't you know?"

"It looks like one on the CT scan, but you never can be completely sure until you operate and have tissue to inspect in the pathology lab. We're about 90 to 95 percent sure."

"Tell me a bit about the family," asks Reverend Carlisle.

"He's a resident in obstetrics," you reply.

"He's a rude, arrogant, self-centered SOB!" chimes in the head nurse. "He's thoughtless, cold, and cares nothing for other people. I wouldn't tolerate him for my doctor and I'm glad I'm not married to him. He walks all over his wife; she's not part of their decisions at all. All Mrs. Peters has done since Monica was admitted is cry. I think that she's afraid to express an opinion and too overwhelmed to think for herself. Monica is their only child."

"Well, let me see," says Reverend Carlisle. "Before we discuss what should be decided, let's consider who should decide. Traditionally, it is the parents' right to decide what is best for their child. They are closest to the child and the ones most likely to have her best interest in mind, so long as they are making an informed decision."

"That's all well and good," says Mary, Monica's primary nurse, "but they also have the most to lose if she survives. This egocentric bastard only wants to make his mark in academic medicine. He doesn't want to be burdened or distracted by a sick child around the house. That just might force him to come home at a reasonable hour, to spend some time with his poor wife, or at least to feel guilty about not doing so. I don't believe for a minute that he's looking out for what's best for Monica. He's looking for what's most convenient for himself!"

"Those are pretty harsh words, young lady. Do not judge lest ye be judged. What would you decide if she were your daughter?"

Mary is somewhat taken aback. She thinks for a time. "Well, first, I would want to be sure that the doctors had the correct diagnosis, so I'd go through with the operation and removal of as much of the tumor as possible. If it is a medulloblastoma, I think I'd probably go along with the chemotherapy and wait on radiation to see how she did. I think quality of life is as important as quantity, so I'd take a somewhat lower survival rate to avoid the retardation from radiation."

"That's fine for you to say, Mary, but you aren't the one dying because your parent is worried you might be dumb. Even a 10-percent chance of survival is good—infinitely better than giving her no chance. Of course, she has to have the operation, even if we have to go to court. There's a 1-percent chance that this could be something odd and totally benign. The operation would cure it. If, however, it does turn out to be a medulloblastoma, we would still have to give her our best shot with radiation. Then she has at least a 50-percent chance of not being retarded. Later, if there's a recurrence, perhaps we can decide not to do something heroic. But at the moment we are talking about only usual and ordinary care for diagnosis and initial therapy. It's what we give every other child who comes here. Doctors' children shouldn't get special treatment." Andrew, the new intern, believes strongly in egalitarian medicine and is eager to treat every baby and everything.

"I'd agree with you, Andy, if this was an older child," interrupts the other resident. "If it were an adolescent or adult I'd strongly urge them to go for it, but Monica's only 2 years old. She doesn't know what life's all about. For her it's about what happens every day, not about the future. What will happen each day is needles, hospitals, discomfort, and separation from mommy and daddy. It's about vomiting from medication and hair falling out—it's about being sick. All this for a small chance at a future she doesn't know or think about. I don't know what I'd decide, but I can easily understand letting her die soon and avoid all of these problems."

"So can I," says the head nurse, "but that is not why Dr. Peters doesn't want the operation. He can't stand sick or dying kids around him. He told me that it was because of children like this that he went into obstetrics. He wants to deal with happy parents and well babies. He's not looking out for Monica; he's looking out strictly for himself. Aren't the motives behind a decision as important as the decision itself?"

"Hmm," responds Reverend Carlisle. "It seems we have a situation where some of us want to do everything and some are willing to do nothing, but none of us are willing to allow Dr. Peters to decide because we don't like the basis for his decision. Is that right? Well, he *does* have the right to decide. If we disagree with his decision, then either we would have to convince him of the "correct" decision, whatever that is, or we would have to feel strongly enough to go to court."

"Before we get too upset, let's wait until he's spoken with Dr. Longsworth this afternoon. Dr. Longsworth's been at this game a long time; I'm sure he'll get Dr. Peters to make the right decision. Let me know if I can be of further help."

*   *   *

Whose decision is this anyway? Is it yours as the resident taking care of Monica? Is it Dr. Longsworth's as the responsible physician and chairman of the department? Is it the parents' decision? Paternalism often seems to be a dirty word. Is it always objectionable? Are parents who act in the best interests of the child being paternalistic? Does anyone other than the child's parents have the right to be paternalistic? As a physician, do you have the responsibility to prevent the parents from making a wrong decision? As an arbiter of right and wrong, can you avoid being paternalistic? Since Dr. Peters has done extensive research on Monica's condition and knows the possible outcome of therapy, how could you justify forcing treatment?

How should the parents' motivation enter into your thinking about what should be done? Would it be proper not to operate if you were convinced that the parents were deciding for Monica's benefit? Would the same decision be wrong if it was made primarily for the parents' benefit? How do you know what the parents' motivation is? Are you qualified to assess that motivation? What approach to morality are you using to judge that motivation? Are you applying the same standards to the motivation of a staff member?

Think about which decision you would make and which decision you would tolerate others making. What principle would you use to define the limits of your tolerance?

Once you have thought about these issues, continue.

Doctor Longsworth's Office

"It's a pleasure to finally meet you, Dr. Longsworth. Monica's mother and I have decided not to go through with the operation. In view of the outlook for Monica, there seems little point in putting her through the pain and suffering. Your staff and residents have been very kind. We'd like to take her home this afternoon. It's best if she dies comfortably."

Dr. Longsworth looks like Dr. Welby of television fame. Kindly, gray haired, with a soft Southern accent, he has been the senior staff surgeon at Metropolitan for the past 10 years.

"Well, son," he drawls, "that's a rough way to meet your patient's family. I understand how you must feel. You put all your eggs in one basket; it dropped and they just broke. However, don't you think we should see if there might be at least one that's still whole? Maybe we could salvage something. How would you feel if Monica died and at autopsy we found that this tumor was benign? Granted, there's not much of a chance of it, but her chances are zero if we don't look. You know, if I had a little girl like Monica I wouldn't want to see her suffer either, and it would break my heart to see her retarded. But suppose the tumor was benign and we could remove it and cure her—that's what we all would really want. I think we should give her that chance, that tiny chance. We can take this one decision at a time. If it is a medulloblastoma, we'll do what we can at surgery and afterward decide about the pro's and con's of radiation or chemotherapy.

"You think about it. I won't take her off the operation schedule just

17

yet. She's on for 7:30 tomorrow morning. Call me at home tonight; otherwise I'll see you in the waiting room tomorrow."

* * *

Before continuing, look at this from different perspectives. If you were Monica's parent, would you allow the operation? Why? Because it gives her the best chance for survival? Because the tumor might be benign? Because Dr. Longsworth has made you feel guilty if you didn't give consent, and guilt is even harder for you to tolerate than your child's suffering or death?

Look at it from the resident's viewpoint. Suppose the parents refuse the operation. Would you tolerate that decision? Would you go to court? Do you think you would win in court?

Think about who should make such a decision and why either decision might be made. How do you evaluate motivation behind decisions? What weight do you give to those motivations? Are you being paternalistic? Can you avoid it? Is paternalism good or bad?

Do you think that by emphasizing the remote chance that the tumor is benign, Dr. Longsworth is manipulating the parents? Is such manipulation good or bad? Is it a legitimate tactic?

If you think that the parents will be swayed by Dr. Longsworth's arguments and will allow the operation, turn to the section "The Operation Was Performed" (p. 20).

If you believe the parents will refuse the operation, you have two options: If you will go to court, turn to the next section. If you will acquiesce and allow them to take Monica home, turn to the section "No Operation Is Performed" (p. 19).

You Go to Court

The operation was canceled, and the hospital's lawyers drew up the papers at Dr. Longsworth's request. They stated Monica's condition and the need for urgent surgery. Dr. Peters presented his side very emotionally and very well. He cited the literature frequently, noting case reports on the poor quality of life of the survivors. It was a tense time in the judge's chambers. The question, however, seemed to revolve around the issue of whether a 20-percent chance of survival was a big number or a small number, especially when there was a 50-percent chance of retardation or other neurologic deficit. Dr. Longsworth and Dr. Peters had very different opinions about that.

* * *

What do you think is a sufficiently reasonable chance to require surgery, 20, 10, or 5 percent? Where would you draw the line? On what basis would you decide?

What do you think the judge will decide? Flip a coin to see what the decision will be. If the coin comes up heads, turn to "The Operation Was Performed" (p. 20). If the coin comes up tails, continue with the following section.

No Operation Is Performed

It's now four months since Monica went home from the hospital. Once the decision was made not to operate, there was no reason for her to stay. In addition, the staff was so upset they recommended that the Peters' find a new physician. The parents took Monica home and are providing her with loving care. It is not easy. Monica is less responsive and vomits frequently because of the increased intracranial pressure. She has lost 10 pounds, is not alert, and cannot see because the pressure in her head has also caused blindness. She no longer seems to be suffering; she just lays there, unresponsive. She must be fed by a tube through her nose. Mrs. Peters has also lost weight and looks physically and emotionally exhausted. She told the ward nurse, who has kept in contact, that she "only hopes it comes soon." Her husband will be back from the obstetrics meetings in Chicago on Friday.

* * *

Was this a good outcome? For whom? It certainly will not be a relatively quick and painless death for Monica. Review your decisions. Would you rather have done the operation? Justify your decisions in moral terms. If, on reconsideration, you would have made different decisions, go back and start again. In the safe confines of this book, you can have more than one chance to get it right.

The Operation Was Performed

Monica has done well in the four days since surgery. The medulloblastoma could not be completely removed. Dr. Peters is considering whether to allow the team to begin chemotherapy next week. He is still not happy about the potential outcome.

On rounds this morning the intern reports that Monica has just spiked a temperature of 103°F. Her spinal fluid shows evidence of meningitis, probably acquired at the time of the operation.

"Of course we'll treat her meningitis," you respond. "That's no big deal. You start the IV while I write the orders. Mary, do we have Ampicillin and Gentamicin on the ward? If not, call the pharmacy. We can finish rounds in a few minutes."

"No needles," Monica cries, then screams, but the IV is rapidly inserted and taped down. Her hands are restrained.

"Has Dr. Peters decided about chemotherapy?" asks the head nurse.

"Not yet," you reply. "He still seems to be against it, but lots of people have been talking to him. I think he'll come around. We wouldn't want to start chemotherapy until next week, anyway. There has to be sufficient time for the wound to heal."

"You know, something bothers me," says the medical student. "We've spent hours talking about whether or not to give chemotherapy to this little girl, about who has the right to make that decision, and the basis for the decision, then this morning you diagnose meningitis and start treatment. No discussion; you didn't even ask the father. Isn't treatment for meningitis a moral issue? If not, why not? If the best thing for Monica is not to treat her tumor and not to prolong her suffering, why are we treating her meningitis? Wouldn't that be a quick way for her to die?"

* * *

Should there have been a discussion of treating the meningitis? Is the treatment of meningitis a straightforward medical matter, or is there a moral issue as well? Is the treatment of meningitis so routine that it is ordinary care and therefore morally required? Or are there circumstances in which the treatment of meningitis becomes extraordinary care, that is, a situation in which treatment is optional and not morally required? What medical factors make treatment either ordinary or extraordinary? Are there nonmedical factors involved in this distinction? Do you always have to discuss the initiation or discontinuation of fluid therapy, feeding, blood tests or respirator care?

Monica

If every medical decision has a significant moral component, requiring extensive discussion, would physicians and nurses have time to care for patients instead of discussing the issues?

*   *   *

That afternoon Monica is found to be anemic, and you order a transfusion. The anemia may be due to the loss of blood at the operation or to the effects of the infection. You also find some blood in the stool, so she might be developing an ulcer, caused by all the stress. After the blood transfusion is started, you check your other patients, sign out to the coresident who is covering you, and go home for the weekend.

At 6 A.M. Saturday the night nurse checks Monica and finds she has vomited a large amount of blood. Monica is pale and has a weak pulse. The nurse puts in a STAT (emergency) page for the resident on the intensive care unit (ICU) and for the resident who is covering for you. Quick assessment reveals that Monica is in shock from a bleeding ulcer. The residents have her immediately transferred to the ICU, order blood from the blood bank, and increase the rate of IV fluid.

One of the residents calls Monica's father at home to tell him of the situation. His reply is, "Don't do anything! I've decided not to put her through any more suffering. She should not be resuscitated. I'll be there within an hour."

*   *   *

What should the ICU resident do now? He does not know Monica or her father. He has heard a bit about the case, but he has not been involved in the discussions, nor has the coresident covering Monica. He checks the chart, but there is no DNR (do not resuscitate) order written.

Consider what you would do if you were in his position. Your decision may make the difference between whether Monica lives or dies. You will have anywhere from a minute to an hour or more to decide. Monica could have a cardiac or respiratory arrest at any moment from the blood loss. Would you resuscitate her? Against her father's wishes? She urgently needs a blood transfusion. Would you begin it or wait for her father?

If there has already been a decision *not* to give her chemotherapy or radiotherapy, why do you want to intervene in a situation that would probably allow her to die quickly? Since you have not been her treating resident up to this point, do not know the background, and have not worked with the family, does this affect your decision? Which way—toward being more vigorous or toward less intervention? Has the decision *not* to give chemotherapy been made? By whom? Is it a reasonable decision?

While you are considering these issues, the blood bank calls to tell you that the blood is ready. Monica still appears to be in shock. Her father is still 30 to 45 minutes away. You will have to decide whether to start the transfusion or wait for her father's arrival.

Before you do, reflect on whether this emergency decision is different from the original decision about operating. If it is different, why? Is it influenced by the fact that you are an outsider to the case? Would you make a different decision if you had been caring for Monica all along and been involved in the dilemma?

If you decide *not* to begin the transfusion, continue with the following section. If you decide to begin the transfusion, turn to "Monica Is Transfused" (p. 23).

Monica Is Not Transfused   You decide to call Dr. Longsworth, and he says he will be right in. He advises you not to start the transfusion unless things get much more critical. Fortunately, nothing worse happens.

Drs. Longsworth and Peters arrive about the same time. After a long discussion, Dr. Longsworth acknowledges that with the very poor outlook, he cannot and will not force the issue again. He established the diagnosis and, to a large extent, the prognosis by finding the medulloblastoma and being unable to remove it totally.

While this discussion is winding down, the nurse shouts that Monica has vomited a large amount of blood. You rush in and find that she has no heartbeat. No resuscitation is attempted, and Monica is declared dead.

Is this a good outcome? For whom? It certainly was a relatively quick and painless death for Monica. Review your decisions. Would you rather have not done the operation? Would you rather have transfused her? Justify your decisions in moral terms. If, on reconsideration, you would have made different decisions, go back and start again. In the confines of this book, you can have more than one opportunity to get it right.

Monica Is Transfused   You begin the transfusion and the blood is running well. Monica is looking pinker; her pulse is stronger and slower. Dr. Longsworth arrives on the ward for his early morning rounds; hearing that Monica has been transferred to the ICU, he comes directly there. You fill him in on what has been happening and tell him that Dr. Peters should be in at any minute.

"Thanks for taking such good care of Monica," says Dr. Longsworth. "You know, one of the nice things about working in a teaching hospital is that we have such good residents who make all the tough decisions in the middle of the night and let us old duffers get our rest. Now, son, what do you think we should do about Dr. Peters? I've been thinking we've been pretty hard on that boy. Maybe he's right. Maybe we're just pressing too hard for Monica. Maybe she'd be best up with those other angels instead of suffering the tortures we put these kids with brain tumors through. We've shown that it isn't a curable tumor. We'd just be putting her through more agony. . . ."

Dr. Peters arrives just then. He sees the blood transfusion running and is about to explode with anger when Monica vomits a large amount of blood. You look at the heart monitor, and her heart has stopped.

Is this a good outcome? For whom? It certainly was a relatively quick and painless death for Monica. Review your decisions. Would you rather have not done the operation? Justify the decisions you made in moral terms. If, on reconsideration, you would have made different decisions, go back and start again. In the confines of this book, you can have more than one chance to get it right.

Chapter 3

LeRoy

"LeRoy, I think it's time we fixed those cataracts. They're getting kind of bad. Making it sort of hard for you to find the young ladies, I imagine?"

"Yes, sir. Can't find the ladies no more, and the rheumatism makes it hard for me to chase 'em. 'Tain't like the old days, no sir. When you get to be my age, things just ain't the same."

"How old are you now, LeRoy?"

"Eighty-three."

"Really? You look more like 75. If it weren't for your eyes and that rheumatism, I'd bet you'd be back swinging a hammer on the railroad. How'd you like to get one of those eyes fixed next week?"

"Yes, sir, that'd be mighty fine."

"Well, I'll set it up. You have someone bring you up here at 8 A.M. on Tuesday. Remember, no breakfast for you; we can't operate if you eat. We'll do the operation about 10 A.M., and you can go home in the late afternoon. You'll have to be careful about the eye and have it checked every few days. Then you'll be better than ever."

"How long will I be in the hospital, Doc? I have to see if I can find someone to look after my dog and the chickens."

"You're not going to be in the hospital at all, LeRoy. The way we do these things now, you don't need it, and the new Medicare rules say they won't pay for a hospital stay. Patients just come in and go out the same day. That's why you need someone to bring you up here and take you home and look after you for a few days until we get the bandages off your eye."

"Who's that gonna be, Doc?"

"Who's what?"

"That person who's gonna bring me here and look after me?"

"Don't you have someone—your wife, children, a friend?"

"No, sir. My wife died 20 years ago. Only had one son and he died in the war. Got a sister, Carolyn, but she's in Oklahoma City. Haven't seen her since my wife died, and Carolyn's got a bad heart. Friends—I've been to more funerals than I can remember. Gets kinda lonely when you get to be my age, Doc. There's just me and Rusty and the chickens. Don't you worry about me, Doc, I'll be here. I'll just catch the 5:30 bus up here in the morning like I always do and take the 6:30 bus back to the farm in the evening. I been looking after myself for a long time, Doc. I'll be fine."

"Where do you live, LeRoy?"

"I got a little piece of land over by Odenville—'bout 30 miles from here. Little house we built a long time ago—grow my vegetables, have a few chickens, and Rusty. Yes, sir, we do fine. Get my railroad check and social security every month—'bout $250. When those chickens is laying good, get another $25. Got my own vegetables, couple of pigs—I'm doing just fine. You fix those eyes, then I won't be missing the eggs and it'll be even better. Don't worry 'bout me, Doc."

"Just a minute, LeRoy, I've got to talk with someone. I don't like the idea of sending you back home alone on the bus with one eye bandaged and no one to look out for you. We used to keep people in the hospital for a couple of days after this kind of surgery just to get over the anesthesia and make sure everything was okay. These new Medicare rules have changed things, but let me see what I can do."

"Is this the admitting office? Mrs. Cleary? What are the rules about admitting someone for cataract surgery? I have this 83-year-old gentleman, living by himself on a farm 30 miles away—bad arthritis, so it's hard for him to get around, and no family or friends to help. I can't send him home the same day as his operation. I'd like him admitted for three days."

"Is he on Medicare, Doctor?"

"Yes."

"I'm sorry, Medicare will not pay for the admission. They have determined that his surgery can be done as an outpatient. Does he have other insurance?"

"I doubt it."

"Could he pay for the room? It's $275 per day."

"I doubt it."

"Well, I'm sorry, but I don't know what we can do. Perhaps if you called Mr. Ball, the hospital administrator, he might have a solution for you. His extension is 8275."

"Mr. Ball? This is Dr. Klein in Ophthalmology. I have this 83-year-old. . . . That's just not right, Mr. Ball. LeRoy just happens to be poor. He's really done very well for himself. He makes it on his own, and now, just because he's poor, he can't get the care he needs. Suppose he falls getting off the bus on the way home or stumbles over something in the house when he can only partially see out of one eye? Aren't we legally responsible? Shouldn't we be morally responsible? You mean to say that this hospital couldn't afford to write off $750 to $1000 on his hospital bill? You'd make him pay it out of his $250 monthly income?" "Yes, I suppose he could go to the public hospital; it's only 300 miles away!"

"Dr. Klein, calm down," responds Mr. Ball. "I understand why you're irate. Believe me, I'm irate, too. I didn't go into hospital administration to protect hospitals from patients. I want to help people, too. I've been through this with so many committees here at the hospital, at the county and state levels, and with the federal administration that I guess my anger's just worn out. Of course, the hospital could write off $1000. Two days ago, I had a call from a physician in gynecology asking about someone else with a problem; we wrote off $2000. I have a message to call the head of pediatrics, who's probably going to ask for something similar. Community Memorial Hospital doesn't have unlimited resources to write off bad debts. If we don't conserve our endowment, we won't have the facilities to provide the care you and I want to give patients. That's why I've been assigned the role of gatekeeper. The new HMO in town is skimming off the paying patients and referring those who can't pay to us. When I talk to the Medical Assistance and Medicare people in the capitol, they say they're in a bind, too. Washington is giving them less money with which to work. The state legislature hasn't raised taxes to take up the slack as federal programs are cut. In this recession they have less money and we have more needy patients. Maybe things are going back to where they were 30 years ago when there were two classes of medical care: the rich get one class and the poor another, or none at all. I don't like it, but I don't see what we can do.

"Officially, I'm going to tell you that you can admit him, but we will have to bill him for those three days. Unofficially, I'll tell you that if he sends you the bill and you bring it to me, I'll write it off. Remember, I never told you this. I can't do it very often or for very many physicians or we'll be broke, so please don't tell anyone. And if you know any congressmen perhaps you can get them to help this country get its priorities straight once again. Have a good day."

* * *

Perhaps you'd like to write to your congressman, outlining the problem. How would you like to see the priorities structured? Remember that the LeRoys of the world and their need for medical care must compete with welfare, food stamps, the farmers and their plight, fire fighters and police, education and, on a national level, social security, defense and myriad entitlements and other social programs. They all have to be paid for by someone, with taxes now or debt, which means taxes later. Your congressman wants to be reelected, and increased taxes are not a popular platform.

Think about the macroallocation of finite resources and their impact on society, on the country as a whole, on the state and its needs, on your county and its obligations, on the hospital, and on LeRoy. Use ethical theories to further your arguments. Indicate to your congressman a more equitable approach to this allocation.

Chapter 4

Joey, Jessica, Roger, Tom, and Marti

It is a beautiful Memorial Day weekend, which means trouble for you. As a fellow in intensive care medicine at University Hospital, you know it is going to be tough. There will be automobile accidents, boating accidents, plus all the usual problems. Since University is the pediatric intensive care center for the entire state, you know you will be busy.

Indeed, as you sign in with the ICU ward clerk at 8 A.M. on Saturday, you see from the patient board that every bed is occupied. This means that even at the beginning of the weekend you are on "flyby." The helicopters that bring injured children to major medical centers now have an order to bypass University for the less well equipped regional centers. The regional centers are not bad; they can handle 90 percent of the cases. However, there is that 10 percent that only the staff and facilities at University can handle really well.

You are especially concerned about the victims of near drownings. University has a special project in this area, and you, the residents, and nurses with whom you work have developed into a team for handling these cases. The team has had excellent results. Children who would have died elsewhere walk out of University with minimal damage. The outcome from many other centers may even be worse—an irreversible coma preceding a lingering death. Although not many people will be swimming today, there will be a lot of boating on the lake. The water is still cold, and that is good for preserving brain function. If someone were to get in trouble, you would have an excellent chance of helping them.

You join the rest of the team in the conference room and begin a review of the patients. Most of the review is just the daily update on each patient's condition. But you and the rest of the staff are anxious to see if

28

one or two patients could be moved out to make room for any disaster that might happen. Here are the patients whom at least one member of the staff thinks are good candidates for leaving the ICU.

Joey

Joey is the kid wearing the Milwaukee Brewers cap and sleeping peacefully in the far corner of room B. Joey has been that way for six months now, and he will never wake up. His brain was severely damaged when his mother's boyfriend, in a drunken stupor, knocked him around the room. The resulting skull fracture and concussion built up such pressure in his head that most of the blood flow through his brain was cut off. His entire cortex, the seat of all the higher functions of the brain, was destroyed by the lack of oxygen. Only a few of his brainstem functions remain. He withdraws from deep pain; if his upper arm muscles are pinched hard, he tries to pull away. His pupils narrow when a light is shined in his eyes. If a cotton swab is brushed across the back of his throat, he gags. He exerts some effort to breathe, but he is now on a respirator because he does not exert enough respiratory effort to sustain himself. If he were disconnected from the respirator, he would gasp for air and, without assistance, would soon suffocate.

This will be Joey's fate. His mother was unwilling to accept it for a long time, especially because the charge against her boyfriend will be changed from assault to murder. Slowly and grudgingly she has come to see that Joey's condition is incurable and that the respirator is merely keeping him breathing. The Child Abuse Agency of the Department of Social Services finally accepted it as well, reluctantly agreeing to get a court order to allow University to discontinue useless therapy; as Joey's guardians, no decision could be made without them, and they took a long time making up their minds. Because Joey's injury is the basis for a criminal prosecution, the district attorney also had to approve withdrawing the respirator. She took only a week to decide that withdrawing the respirator would not damage her case for a murder conviction.

It took three months to stabilize Joey's condition and to be sure that he had suffered irreversible brain damage. It took the second three months to put the pieces of a decision together. Wednesday of this week, everyone was in court reviewing the entire case before Judge McBrien. He heard everyone out, asked a number of questions of the physicians about how sure they were that Joey would not recover (they were very sure), and announced that he would hand down his decision in a week. The hospital's attorneys assured the ICU team that there would be no problem, that Judge McBrien would let them withdraw the respirator. They cautioned, however, that the judge did not like being rushed and that he liked his weekends off. There was nothing to do, the attorneys advised, but wait one more week.

Joey's fate, then, was decided, but you are powerless to do anything about it. If you turn the respirator off before the judge hands down his order, you and the hospital could be guilty of contempt of court. Worse, you would never again get a sympathetic hearing from Judge McBrien or other judges if you needed a decision in a similar case.

The only other possibility is to move Joey to another ward in the hospital. But there are problems here as well. Hospital policy is very clear on the point: no pediatric respirator patients outside the ICU. The policy is based on some bad past experiences. Furthermore, since the staff on other wards had lost touch with the care of respirator patients, there is the risk that Joey might die outside the ICU. That might not sit well with the judge, and who knows what effect it would have on the prosecution of Joey's assailant.

As you run through these considerations with the team, there is a growing sense of frustration and anger. Who are we treating, they ask, Joey or the lawyers? We did absolutely everything we could for Joey, and it did not work. For the last three months, all we have been doing is torturing him while everyone goes to meetings. Now we are not only torturing Joey, but we are going to find ourselves turning away some child we could really help. This is an abuse of everything the ICU stands for; it is immoral unless we can free up Joey's bed or some other bed in the ICU.

You agree, but what can you do? You go on to the next case.

Jessica

Jessica, like Joey, will soon be out of the ICU, but her story will have a happy ending. Jessica has Guillain-Barre syndrome, an inflammation of the nervous system that sometimes follows a viral infection. The disease causes a progressive paralysis, starting in the hands and feet and proceeding to the trunk. It is usually self-limiting and self-reversing. In 90 percent of the cases, the disease is not recurrent and there are no long-term effects. When the disease affects the trunk, however, the muscles of the chest become paralyzed and the patient cannot breathe on her own. These patients are placed on respirators until their nerve functions return and their muscles regain normal strength.

Jessica has been in the ICU for about two weeks, and she is doing very well. The paralysis seems to be improving, and she is starting to recover. Her respiratory muscles have not regained full strength, so she still needs some support from a respirator. It will be about two weeks before she can be taken off it entirely.

As in Joey's case, hospital policy requires that Jessica stay in the ICU. Unlike Joey's, the quality of medical care will have a bearing on the outcome of her case. If someone on another ward makes a mistake in handling Jessica, even though it would be difficult to make such a mistake because her care is relatively simple at this point, Jessica could suffer brain damage or even die. The nurse who has been working most closely with Jessica is adamant.

"There is no way Jessica is going anywhere else. I know she doesn't need a great deal of care at this moment, but no one else in this hospital is competent to provide that care. It would simply be immoral to transfer Jessica to another ward. We can't take that chance on a child who is doing so well.

"Furthermore, if you want to talk hospital policy and legal problems, what kind of shape would we be in if something happened to Jessica? Her father is a lawyer, and he was very upset when their local pediatrician didn't make the diagnosis right away. If we try anything less than standard medical care, all hell will break loose."

The resident in charge of the near-drowning resuscitation group now spoke up.

"It just isn't true that Jessica's care off this ward would be substandard. The hospital's policy on respirator patients is very artificial, especially in a case like this when Jessica doesn't require that much. We even send kids home on respirators. It is crazy that we can't send them to another unit in this hospital. We would have to hunt up a nurse with some respirator experience, or even send one of you down to check on things, but Jessica will do just fine. In the meantime, we would be able to help someone for whom the ICU is a life-or-death matter. Right now Jessica requires chronic care. She is not an intensive care patient. We don't have to move her before we have another patient, of course, but I think she is the logical one to go if the need arises."

In Joey's case, the team had been pretty much of one mind. The ICU was not doing anything for Joey, but the legal risks of moving him out were very high. In Jessica's case, there was a division of opinion among the staff, so you thought it best to move on.

31

Roger

Roger is dead. He committed suicide on Thursday night by putting his father's revolver in his mouth and firing. From the time he was brought to the emergency room, it was clear there was no hope. It was also clear that he was an ideal organ donor. Roger was placed on a respirator immediately and treated to insure the survival of his kidneys and liver. The neurology resident examined him on Friday and agreed that all clinical signs said that Roger was dead. He had no gag reflex, made no effort to breathe when temporarily disconnected from the respirator, and made no response to pain. An electroencephalogram (test of brain waves) showed a tiny amount of activity. A second test ordered for today will undoubtedly show no activity. The neurologists will declare Roger dead whenever you want.

Yesterday was very hard. Although Roger had previously shown signs of what is now recognized as depression, he had no prior history of mental illness and had never threatened suicide. His parents are completely devastated. The nurses and a psychiatrist spent all day yesterday with them. His parents slowly and painfully came to accept Roger's death and even raised the possibility of his being an organ donor. It was a way that some part of him would remain alive; even in death he would make some contribution. They signed the papers last evening.

Meanwhile, the hospital's own transplant group was alerted. After doing blood and tissue typing on Roger, they identified him as a heart donor for one of their patients. The liver transplant team in a nearby state was notified, and they had a suitable recipient. They were gearing up, and a group would fly in late today to pick up Roger's liver. The kidney transplant group was also preparing two recipients.

The plan was to take Roger to an operating room in the early evening. He would be declared dead, the respirator would be removed, and the organs would be taken for transplant. Until then, Roger would stay on the respirator and on his blood pressure medications to keep his organs in shape. Nothing could be done before early evening because it would take at least that long for the transplant teams to get ready.

"I think Roger is the one who should go," says the head nurse. "He's dead. He is no longer a patient. No matter what shape the others are in, they are our patients and we are committed to doing what is best for them, even if, in Joey's case, it means doing little or nothing. These transplant patients are not ours. It will be a shame if they do not get Roger's organs, but that's not our problem. We have to keep our eyes on what we're doing here, not looking out for everyone else's problems."

"That's a good point," volunteered the resident who was directing the near-drowning project; another resident reminded the group that the people coming in on helicopters aren't their patients either.

"Not exactly right," the nurse replied. "We have a special state grant to operate the resuscitation program. We've trained the helicopter crews. Once drowning victims are picked up, they are our patients. As part of the state program, we have a responsibility for them."

You raise the point that the team may have a responsibility to Roger, even though he is dead. Yesterday you made a commitment to accept his organs for donation. That means a lot to his parents and might even mean something to him had he been aware of it. Besides, you add, perhaps the crunch will not come until tomorrow after all the organ donations have taken place.

"Could we at least transfer him to pediatrics temporarily?" asks one of the residents. "Not if you're serious about maintaining him in decent shape for the next 6 to 8 hours," responds the head nurse. "We have enough problems with the respirator down there; with all Roger's drugs and machines—no way those nurses could handle that. We're already short staffed on the holiday. He needs constant monitoring to keep his blood pressure up. It's almost a full-time job for a nurse."

"Is there any way we could go over census and squeeze an extra bed in here?" you ask.

"Usually we could, but not this weekend. I've cut things to the bone to give staff the weekend off and, on top of that, Nancy called in sick. We'll be lucky to get by as is," says the head nurse.

Your mental list of candidates for non-ICU treatment is exhausted, and you are about to get a cup of coffee and think the thing through when Karen, the pediatric resident, interrupts.

"I think you are skipping over two of the most obvious players," she says. "There are two kids here with chronic conditions that, in my view, are better nominees than any of the three we've been talking about.

"I took an ethics course in college," she continued, "and we talked about cases like this in terms of the allocation of scarce medical resources. It was a question of social ethics and public policy. Our discussion is looking at individual cases too narrowly, taking them out of their social context. The three cases we've talked about so far will be over in a day, or maybe a week. But there are two kids in this unit who have long-term, massive, and very expensive problems. I think we should consider moving them out of the unit because I don't think it's right for society to treat

33

them. For what it's costing to treat these two kids, we could do near-drowning cases for a decade. I'm thinking of Tom and Marti."

Tom

Tom was born about eighteen months ago with prune-belly syndrome. Just before the midpoint of his mother's pregnancy, his urethra became blocked and the urine backed up into his bladder and then into the kidneys. This condition was detected in a routine ultrasound exam at about the twenty-sixth week of pregnancy, and his mother was referred to the obstetrical group at University. Tom's mother was in her middle thirties, a professional woman who had long postponed having a child. Amniocentesis showed Tom to be genetically normal, and she was anxious for any help to continue the pregnancy. In turn, the obstetrical group was anxious to get started on new techniques of in-utero surgery. They persuaded Tom's mother to let them try.

In the twenty-eighth week of the pregnancy, the obstetrical surgeons inserted a catheter through his mother's abdomen into Tom's distended bladder. This shunt drained urine from the bladder into the amniotic fluid, decompressing the kidneys and restoring the normal amniotic fluid volume.

It was one of those "the operation was a success but the patient died" stories, only this patient did not die. Tom was born in the thirty-fourth week of his mother's pregnancy. The pressure on his kidneys was relieved only temporarily. As the volume of amniotic fluid again declined because the shunt stopped working, Tom's mother started premature labor. The obstetricians decided that an early delivery would give Tom the best chance, so they did a Caesarian section.

Tom was born with a grossly distended, wrinkly abdomen—hence the name prune-belly syndrome. In addition, as is common in this condition, his lungs were underdeveloped. Tom was placed on a respirator at birth and could never be removed.

Over the past eighteen months, everything was tried, and nothing worked very well. The damage that Tom's lungs suffered in utero could not be significantly reversed, nor could the kidney damage be reversed, so Tom needs regular dialysis. Moreover, Tom has not done well intellectually or socially. His development has been substantially slow, although there is no clear reason for this. Tom's mother has stuck with him, but it is now clear that he is not developing normally. She is very discouraged about the prospect of what she calls a "reasonable life" for Tom.

"Listen," Karen argued, "we all know now that the obstetricians made a mistake. They never should have tried their fancy new operation; they were just hopping on the bandwagon. Even in the literature then available, there was good reason to think it wouldn't work. But once we got started, no one has been able to say 'stop.' Tom is stable, of course, but none of us is facing the fact that he will never come off the ventilator and that he will never lead what remotely could be called a normal life. His development is very poor, and it isn't going to get any better. I think we should take him off the respirator and let him die."

There was a commotion around the room, and someone said, "We can't do that!"

When the hubbub died down, Karen continued, "That's the whole trouble with these chronic care kids. There's always *mañana,* and no one really faces up to their troubles. We have been mumbling things to Tom's mother, but we've never sat down to confront her with the facts and, worst of all, we've never confronted ourselves with the facts. There never is a good time to make these decisions. We've already made the decision, but we're just not facing it. We talk about weaning him off the respirator, and we know that's a phony. He'll never make it. Somehow or other, we're going to cut back and he's going to die. Let's cut our losses and act now. We have to face up to the fact that our very expensive therapy hasn't worked, and we can no longer afford to keep Tom going, especially because he is going nowhere."

Karen has a good case, and you know it. But you just do not see how the issue can be resolved this weekend. You can't transfer him to pediatrics because of the respirator and the dialysis that's scheduled this weekend. So you just ask Karen to mention the other case she has in mind.

"The other patient we should discontinue treatment on is Marti."

Marti

From a medical point of view, Marti's case is simple and tragic. A 12-year-old, she was riding in her mother's car when it stopped at a light and was rear ended at high speed by a drunk driver. Marti's spinal cord was severed at the C2 level, the very top of the neck. In terms of control, Marti's head was severed from the rest of her body. She is completely paralyzed from the neck down and, therefore, breathes only because she is on a respirator. She is completely unable to move her legs, arms, or head. She talks, of course, and her intellectual ability is completely unaffected.

35

Marti has been in intensive care for about three months. The initial purpose of her stay was to stabilize her condition and to be sure that the spinal cord damage was complete and irreversible. Now she remains in the ICU until she can be transferred to a rehabilitation hospital.

The driver of the car that hit her had no insurance and no assets to help pay for Marti's care. Marti's mother is a single parent with poor health care coverage. Marti's care is now being handled by the state fund for crippled children.

"This is going to sound awful," Karen said, "but I think it is unfair to keep Marti alive at overwhelming expense when that same money could be used to help so many people. The level of medical care she will require is more than society should invest in any one person. In most places in the world, she would have died soon after the accident. We've assessed her condition, and we know just how handicapped she is going to be. This sounds very hard, but we should sedate her and pull the plug." "Today?" you ask. "We could send her down to pediatrics," says one of the residents. "Unlike Jessica," you reply, "she is totally dependent on the respirator. I would not even risk sending her down to the ward; there's no way she would survive even the slightest glitch."

Karen's previous proposal had caused a commotion; this one caused a near riot. People were shouting and pounding the table.

It just showed how attached they'd become to this totally dependent little girl. "What kind of morality is that, Karen?" asks one of the other residents. "You'd turn off the respirator on someone with normal intelligence just because she's physically handicapped?"

"I suppose there's the alternative of moving Tom or Marti down to the ward," you add, "but that still poses the respirator problems. On Monday we should discuss long-term plans for them with social services. Now is the time to get back to work and to hope that the roof doesn't fall in." You head for the door still hoping that you won't have to make any decisions.

Later That Morning

Several hours later the call comes. You are talking with Marti, who is very depressed. She doesn't want to see the psychiatrist any more, and she thinks it would have been better if she had died in the accident. The soccer season is just ending, and her team lost in the finals. "I'll never be able to do anything," she wheezes around the tracheotomy tube in her throat.

Sally, the triage nurse, pages you to the red phone. As you come down the hall, she calls out that it is Mike from the state police rescue unit. He is on a dock in Lake City with two kids who have just been rescued. The red phone connects you directly with him in the helicopter.

"Hey, Doc, you have to make room for these kids. They're great candidates for you. Their boat tipped over and they were only under water for about ten minutes. They are brothers, 7 and 9 years old. Some guys in another boat saw them go in, fished them out, and did some CPR. Both are breathing but cold and unconscious. I radioed Lakeside Community Hospital right away because I knew you were on flyby. Lakeside pleaded with me to have you take them. They have plenty of room but nobody competent with near drowning. I wanted to take a look at the kids and size up the situation, the way you trained us, before calling in. This is a great setup for your new treatments, but sending them to Lakeside is signing their death warrants, or worse. You just *have* to take these kids, Doc."

* * *

You've been over all of the other alternatives and there just aren't any. The only way you could take one or both of the boys is by displacing one or two of your ICU patients.

If you decide to take one or both of the boys, you have about two hours to decide who to displace and to make appropriate arrangements. You can evaluate and stabilize the drowning victims in the emergency room, but within two hours there will have to be room in your ICU.

Write down your tentative decision and a brief justification for your choice. If you decide to displace one or more of the children from the ICU, also explain why you didn't select the others.

Now that you've justified your decision to yourself, try to delineate the basis for your decision so that others can understand.

Reconsidering and Justifying Your Decision

The best and safest thing for each of the ICU patients is to remain in the ICU. Unfortunately, that is also the best place for the boys on the dock. For each child there is an increased risk if they are removed from the ICU or not brought there. How did you just balance the risks and benefits in making your decision?

Ethical theory provides guidelines for making these decisions. Different theories use different bases. Let's try a few.

Quality of Individual Life

Which patients gain the most from being in the ICU? Who will lose the most by being moved out? Who will lose the least? Does Roger have anything to lose? What about Joey and Tom? How about Jessica and Marti? Rank the 5 patients in order of who has the most to lose. Is that a moral basis for deciding who should stay? Where did you rank the boys on the dock? How much do we know about what they have to lose?

Social Utility

Should you look beyond what an individual has to gain or lose and include family, other individuals, and society in your calculations? This is called social benefit analysis, a type of utilitarian theory.

Social benefit analysis tries to add up the total happiness or self-satisfaction of the individual and the happiness and self-satisfaction of all those with whom he is associated and affects. For example, an anencephalic, an infant with no brain, has no capability for experiencing happiness or satisfaction. If he brings no joy to those around him, he has no social utility. If his family derives some pleasure from him, then he has some utility.

Using this type of calculation, rank the children in the ICU.

How did you rank Roger? Does the fact that he's dead mean that he has no individual utility? What about his social utility to the organ recipients? Does this raise his utility above that of Joey? Tom? Jessica? How would you rank Jessica's utility, when she will be a perfectly normal child, against what Roger can accomplish for several others? How about Marti? What is her "utility" score? How many points do you give her for happiness? Is depression a transient state?

Now give a score to the boys on the dock. Where do they fit into your rank order? Do you know enough about them? You don't even know enough to guess at their prognosis. Will they end up like Joey? Or like Jessica?

Write down your rankings of the 7 individuals.

Rights and Obligations

Under this theory there are certain inalienable rights with which an individual is born. Among these are: the right to respect as a person, from which may flow the right to life or at least the right not to be killed; the right to liberty, often used in the political sense, but also including the

38

right not to be interfered with, and the right to control of one's own person. While many philosophers articulate rights in different fashions and while even the preceding three rights overlap and flow from one another, they are basic rights of personhood.

We are born with some rights, and others are acquired by the commitments and contracts made by other individuals in society. The right to vote, for example, is given by the state and may be withdrawn, as with felons; restricted, as with moving; or extended, as it was to 18-year-olds. The right to medical care is a source of debate, but in our society it often flows from a contract or commitment between patient and physician.

Rights incur obligations (obligations may also generate rights). The obligations you have to your ICU patients have generated their rights to medical care.

Are rights absolute and equal? Or do they have varying degrees of magnitude? Can you rank the patients in order of their rights? Does Roger have any rights? Do the transplant recipients have any rights? Does Joey have any rights? Are Joey's rights just legal and not moral? Are moral rights stronger or weaker than legal rights?

Rerank the patients in order of their rights. Compare your list to the other two lists you made. Are they different? Did it help your decision making to rank them this way?

Do the boys on the dock have a right to your care? Is that right greater than that of any of the ICU patients? If so, what will you do about it?

Now list these same patients in terms of the strength of your obligation to each. Do you have an obligation to the boys on the dock? Do you have an obligation to Roger, even though he is dead? Do you have an obligation to Roger's parents, to the transplant teams, and to the potential transplant recipients? Are your obligations to the transplant teams affected by the commitment that your hospital has made to the program? After you have ranked the patients in terms of the strength of your obligations, compare that list with the other lists previously prepared. How are they related to each other? Which list should be used to make a moral decision?

Now make your decision. How will you handle this crisis? Although you have time to carry out your decision, you have little time to actually decide.

Not only is what you do important, but why you do it counts as well. Try, at least in a sketch in your notebook, to justify the decision you have made. Later events may require that you look back at this first decision, and it will be helpful if you have notes about why you decided as you did.

39

1. If you decided to turn down one or both boys, turn to the section entitled "You Turn Down the Drowning Victims" (p. 45).
2. If you have decided to displace Joey, you better discuss this with Judge McBrien first. Turn to the section following this list.
3. If you plan to displace Jessica, at least call her father and tell him why you changed your mind about keeping her in the ICU. Turn to the section entitled "Jessica" (p. 41).
4. If you plan to displace Roger, call his parents. They were waiting to hear from you about the transplants. Turn to "Roger" (p. 43).
5. If you plan to displace Marti, turn to "Marti" (p. 46).
6. If you decide to accept both boys, decide whom to displace and follow the decision to its end; then return to this page and decide on the second displacement.

Joey

After a lengthy effort you finally locate Judge McBrien at his cottage on the lake. The state police found the boat on which he was fishing. The judge does not take kindly to having his weekend disturbed.

You outline the problem to the judge and carefully explain why it is important to turn off Joey's respirator now. Other lives are at stake.

With seeming patience, the judge explains that he has been thinking deeply about the case and that he thinks best when he is on the lake and *undisturbed*. "This is not an easy case," he says. "You realize, of course, that Joey is not brain dead. By legal standards, if you turn off the respirator you will be killing him. I am agonizing over this case because I don't like my cases appealed and my decisions overturned. I'll let you know my final decision on Wednesday. Please don't disturb me again."

*   *   *

If, in the face of your discussion with Judge McBrien, you decide that you better not do anything about Joey, turn back and choose again.

If you decide that, even though you can't turn off the respirator, you can transfer Joey to pediatrics and take a chance, then continue.

*   *   *

You transfer Joey to pediatrics and discuss the case with the residents and nurses there. You emphasize the need for careful monitoring and tell them to call you with any questions or problems. At 1 A.M. Sunday, Joey's respirator became disconnected. The alarm on the machine did not function. At 2 A.M., when the nurse came in to check his vital signs, Joey was dead.

At noon on Sunday, you are called to the offices of the hospital's general counsel. They are, as usual, not happy and are getting ready to go to court tomorrow to break the news to Judge McBrien. They are preparing a memorandum to the judge explaining why the issues placed before him are now moot.

They ask you to write a brief explanation of what happened to Joey and why he was chosen to be removed from the ICU. Incorporate the considerations you made regarding patient's rights and your obligations to your patients as well as any considerations of risk, benefits, and consequences. Also acknowledge any obligations you have to the courts, the legal systems, and Judge McBrien.

After you've finished your explanation, turn to the "Conclusion," (p. 47).

Jessica

You locate Jessica's father in Chicago, where he is working with a client. He comes to the phone breathlessly.

"Is there something wrong? When I left last night Jessie really seemed so much better and happier, we were really beginning to be hopeful. What happened?"

You reassure him that nothing has happened, that you are calling because she is doing so well. You explain about the drowning and the need for room in the ICU. Jessica is clearly making a good recovery. "I am planning to move her and her respirator down to pediatrics. She should do just fine. We'll put her right across from the nurses' station so they can watch her just in case anything happens."

"What do you mean, in case? What could happen? You told me she needs to be in the ICU another two weeks because it was the safest place for someone on a respirator to be."

After much discussion and as much reassurance as you can muster, Jessica's father acquiesces with one condition. "Dr. Dunn is an old buddy of mine from high school days. He is chief of pediatrics. I know he would look out for her best interests. If he says it's okay, I guess it will be. I'll be in to see her when I get back tomorrow."

41

You put down the phone and call Dr. Dunn, whose wife tells you that he has just left for an international congress in Germany. "Can I help? Dr. Dunn has left that nice young man, Brian, in charge. Why don't you try him?"

Your friend Brian is chief resident in pediatrics. You call him; his response is just what you would expect. "I feel for you, buddy. Two drowning victims, and such a beautiful weekend; you'll never get out for tennis. Sure we'll take her. I'll square it with our head nurse. She doesn't mind bending the rules a bit. Sounds like Jessica shouldn't be a problem. It's a good thing Dunn's out of town—he's pretty rigid about those things. I'll be on the tennis courts if you can get away."

* * *

If you decide to take Brian's offer, continue reading this section. But if you are concerned about not getting Dr. Dunn's permission, as Jessica's father had insisted, go back to the list on page 40 and choose again.

* * *

Jessica came out of it fine; you are confident that she suffered no permanent damage. But Dr. French, the chief of Critical Care Medicine, is standing there with a blank incident report form. You had Jessica moved to pediatrics. They put her in the front room, directly across from the nurses' station, so the staff could keep a close watch on her. Unfortunately, they got so nervous about their first respirator patient in years that they kept looking in on her. They just could not leave her alone. Finally, someone decided that the respirator was not set correctly; Jessica was breathing for herself in between the actions of the machine. (Of course, this was what you wanted. It was part of the process of weaning her from the respirator.) So the first-year resident on duty that night set the machine up to keep pace with her spontaneous respirations. Jessica had adjusted to the reduced use of the machine, and its stepped-up pace shook her out of a sound sleep. The pacing of the machine was very uncomfortable for her, and she whined and thrashed around all night. When you checked on her first thing in the morning, you found an exhausted and very unhappy young patient. A night of utterly foolish activity had probably set her recovery back by several days.

"In the incident report," Dr. French says, "you should explain what a respirator patient was doing outside the ICU, the only unit in the hospital approved for such patients. Tell them why you chose Jessica and explain the relative risks, benefits, and obligations that went into your decision."

When you finish this report, turn to the "Conclusion" on page 47.

Roger

Roger's folks have been waiting for your call. "Have they done the transplants yet?" is their first question. "It's been a rough few days for us, Doctor. But you know, allowing Roger to give of himself really has helped us to come to terms with this. Can you tell us anything about the person who will receive the heart?"

This makes it difficult for you to start. "Well," you begin, "there's a problem. We have these two boys who just fell in the lake, and we're the only hospital that could save them. They're on their way by helicopter, and we need to make room in the ICU. Roger's already dead—we can save the boys. We just wanted you to know why Roger won't be used for a transplant."

"Oh," comes the sinking word. "Dr. Hammill convinced us of the good Roger would bring these others. He sounded as though this new transplant program would really be able to help people. Does he know your plan? We'd like to talk with him."

You barely hang up when the nurse tells you that Dr. Hammill is on the other phone.

"You're going to do what!" is about the only repeatable part of what Dr. Shearson Hammill said. He is head of the heart transplant group and organ donation coordinator for University Hospital. His group has by now started preparing the heart transplant patient for surgery, and a physician and two technicians from the liver transplant group in another city are already in flight. The kidney and cornea groups in the hospital are well along in their preparations.

"All of these preparations are in progress," he screams. "This young boy who's going to receive the heart has been waiting for a donor for four months now. If we don't use Roger's heart, he's not going to make it. The television stations are coming to our press conference this afternoon. And what about my friends from State who have given up their weekend to fly here to get the liver? I've got to work with them in the future, too! If you turn off the respirator and screw things up, you'll hear from the chairman of the board himself! Mr. Stone is personally responsible for getting us this transplant program. It's going to make this hospital's reputation. I'm warning you. . . ."

*   *   *

43

After considering your obligations and commitments to Roger, to his mother, to the transplant recipients, and to Dr. Hammill, if you decide not to turn off the respirator return to the list on page 40 and choose again. If you decide to turn off the respirator anyway, continue reading this section.

* * *

It's a gray Tuesday morning and you have just been ordered to come to the boardroom to meet with Mr. Stone, who is chairman of the hospital's board. As you enter the boardroom, he hands you the front page of the morning paper. The headlines reads "Transplant Candidate Dies."

"I have here a report from Dr. Hammill, head of our transplant group, describing the events of this past weekend. I am outraged! We are a laughingstock. First we have to cancel the press conference, and now this! What have you done?

"I know you were thinking about saving those two boys—and about the near-drowning program with which you've been working—but that's not all that goes on here at University. We have lots of programs. While we certainly have invested in the near-drowning program, we are even more heavily invested in the heart transplant program. That's why we brought Dr. Hammill here, and it wasn't cheap!

"There are more lives to be saved in organ transplant than you'll ever see in this cold water drowning stuff. You should have looked at the big picture, but you were only looking out for your own program, not for University Hospital.

"But it's not just University Hospital. This has to do with society. Your decision flies in the face of good social policy. It just isn't rational!

"If you thought more lives could be saved by caring for these two drowning victims, you better be prepared to prove it. After all, Roger's heart would have saved one life and his liver another. Other organs, kidneys, corneas, etc., could have added greatly to the quality of other lives. As many as six people could have been helped. That doesn't add up too well against the one or two drowning victims that could possibly be saved, and you don't even know how they'd turn out.

"Before you make another decision like this," he said as he slammed the desk, "you better learn to add. You also better write me something that I can use to justify this mess before the Board of Trustees next week!"

* * *

When you write your report explain why you chose to disconnect Roger from the respirator. Explain why your obligations and commitments to other patients outweighed those to Roger, his mother, and the transplant recipients. Do you have any obligations to the hospital and its program?

When you are finished, turn to the "Conclusion" on page 47.

You Turn Down the Drowning Victims

It is a month since you turned down the two boys who were victims of a boating accident. (Since the problems that arise here are the same whether you turned down one or both boys, the section is written as though you turned down both.) You have just finished a phone call with Dr. Robinson French, director of the Division of Critical Care Medicine and one of your supervisors. He was not happy. He was organizing the application for renewal of your unit's special grant for the resuscitation of near-drowning victims and was preparing the section titled "available beds and other resources."

"In our original grant application," he needlessly reminded you, "we assured the federal government that we had adequate space to handle any foreseeable number of victims. Our ICU was underutilized. Now we turned away two prime candidates for our service. We trained the helicopter medics and set the whole thing up around our unit, and now we're turning people away.

"Even worse," he continued, "do you know how those kids are doing up at Lakeside? Terribly, that's how. The guys on duty in the emergency room that morning were orthopedic surgeons who didn't know beans about resuscitation. They followed the old textbook rules. As a result, the kids are still in a coma and are not likely to wake up.

"And just to cap it all off, I've heard on the grapevine that Lakeside is going to try to compete for this grant money. They're going to argue that they are closer to the scene of most boating accidents, and now they've got more space in their ICU. Although he doesn't have the physicians to support the project, the hospital administrator up there is very shrewd and aggressive.

"I want you to draft out this page of the grant application, explaining why you turned these boys down, why we really should have this grant, and how a mess like this won't happen again. Next time we will juggle things around to take care of patients like this."

Uninviting though it was, it beat out your other writing assignment. The boys' parents were suing the hospital. It was a novel kind of malpractice suit based on the parents' claim that because the hospital had a special grant, all near-drowning victims in its service area were actually its patients. The hospital's lawyers had called last week.

"Sketch out," they said, "your reasons for turning these kids down. You had better make sure there was no other course of action. We are going to argue in court that you had an absolute obligation to every patient in the ICU. We want you to provide the medical and ethical arguments about a physician's duties and obligations to buttress our case. And we do not want to go to court with any of those scarce resources and maximizing benefits arguments. They do not go over well before a jury—they sound like doctors play God. Get us a one-page sketch by next week."

Once you've written your one-page sketch, turn to the "Conclusion" on page 47.

Marti

You persuade pediatrics to take Marti. They are nervous about it, but you assure them that you will provide all the help you can and that you will take Marti back as soon as possible. Marti spends an uneventful Saturday night in pediatrics, and on Sunday morning the unexpected death of a cardiac patient means that she can return to the ICU.

From a medical point of view, this decision works out better than any other. Does that make it the right decision? Or was it just a matter of luck? How does the fact that this choice works out well affect your moral evaluation?

Write an entry for your journal explaining why it made good moral sense to remove Marti from the ICU.

Conclusion

Congratulations! You've muddled through. You've either refused the two boys who will be vegetating at Lakeside Hospital for the indefinite future, or you've made room for one or both of them at the expense of your old friends. Did you at least use a good process for your decision? Are you satisfied using obligations, commitments, risks, and benefits as a basis for your moral decision making?

By the way, if you do not want to face the same problem on July 4th weekend, you better make plans for Tom and Marti.

Chapter 5

Tom Revisited

Four days have passed since what is now referred to as the "Memorial Day Massacre." Everyone in the hospital echoes the sentiment: never again. But it is not long until the Fourth of July, and not a minute too soon to start planning. There is no reason to think that the Memorial Day problems will not recur. Even if the Fourth was not around the corner, both Tom and Marti deserve some long-term planning.

You have passed the word that there are tough decisions to be made on social work rounds this morning. All the regulars, and some irregular attenders, are there. The hospital chaplain, the hospital's new biomedical ethicist, the ICU social worker, and Tom's and Marti's nurses are all there.

"Look, team, we're not going to go through that Memorial Day hassle again. Our mistake was in not planning ahead. Joey's gone, so is Roger. Jessica should be home well before July 4th. Only Tom and Marti may be around. We've got to try and make some plans for them while we have time. That's why I've asked for this meeting.

"Let's start with Tom. What should we plan for him?"

"What's to plan?" asks Bernie, the resident currently caring for Tom. "At the moment, there is nothing we can do for Tom but wait and hope. I'll grant there isn't much hope that Tom's lungs are going to develop, but lung transplants may become more practical. They are already doing heart-lung transplants in adults. Meanwhile, we just do more of what we have been doing. We don't really know why Tom hasn't been developing mentally and socially. We should just do for Tom what we do for every other patient—provide the best medical care we can. That's our plain and simple moral obligation. That is what 2000 years of ethical medicine is all about; I don't understand all the fuss."

"Well, I can tell you what the fuss is about," said Professor Bradstreet, the ethicist. "The problem is really a societal one. We are just hiding behind platitudes if we talk of providing 'the best medical care.' Are you talking about the best technical care, or the best care for Tom? If you are looking at what is best for Tom, we have to look at it in the context of what is best for the family, and what is best for society. You cannot look at these things in isolation.

"Our health care delivery system is in mortal crisis. Unless we do something about its spiraling costs, the whole system will come crashing down around us. Medical intervention in Tom's case has been a health care resources disaster from the very first. Results of in-utero surgery have not been very good, as Tom amply illustrates. The hospital has invested an enormous amount of its own money in Tom's case. More worthwhile expenditures have been passed over because so much money is used to support him."

"I hate to interrupt, Professor Bradstreet," said Jim, the ICU social worker, "but I think all the cost arguments will only cloud the issues. It's not our job to worry about the costs and benefits to society, or even to the hospital. Tom is our concern. I don't buy Bernie's line either; we have to consider Tom's future in making our decision.

"The context of Tom's care has got to be his own and his family's situation. It is not just a technical decision, nor something for society as a whole. Tom's care, it seems to me, is primarily his mother's decision. Since Tom cannot make his own decisions, his mother, Rosa, has the right to make them for him. As long as her decision-making seems appropriate, not medically too far out and not outside society's limits, she should make the decisions.

"It has taken Rosa a long time to get over the optimistic stuff she was being handed by the obstetrical surgeons. During the past several months, however, she seems to be getting more realistic. She is getting discouraged, but there is no way she is ready to throw in the towel. She still hopes her son will make it. If you are thinking of letting Tom die, you'll not get Rosa to agree anytime soon."

"Well, it's not just a matter of waiting for Rosa to come around," put in Barbara, Tom's primary nurse. "Although she certainly has the right to a lot of input, we have to explain Tom's situation to her so that her views are reasonable. And the reasonableness of the decision has to be based on a careful assessment of Tom. Of course, we can keep him going as he is almost indefinitely, but is that really for his benefit? Tom is our first concern. We are concerned about Rosa and about our needs in the ICU. We should consider benefits to science and to society, but these should all be secondary; Tom is our primary concern. We have to make a plan. It doesn't matter who decides, the important thing is that we decide what to do on the basis of what's best for Tom. Once we decide what to do, we can figure out how to do it."

Each character in this vignette proposed an overall approach to dealing with Tom's problem.

1. Bernie, the resident, proposed to stick to the duty of physicians to provide medical care independent of outside considerations.
2. Professor Bradstreet proposes to look at the overall costs and benefits to society in deciding about Tom's continued treatment.
3. Jim, the social worker, holds that Tom's mother has the right to make the decision.
4. Barbara, Tom's nurse, wants to decide what is in Tom's best interest and to set up the decision-making situation so as to produce what is most beneficial for Tom.

Each of these represent different ethical approaches to decision making. Read on to see where each leads you.

Bernie's Approach:
Continued Medical Care

"Bernie, the problem of continuing this kind of care forever is that it never ends. What will you do when Tom develops pneumonia? Provide standard care with antibiotics? What about when he gets a systemic infection with one of the bad bugs that respirator patients always get? Five years from now, when Tom is no longer a cute, somewhat delayed infant, but a very retarded child, will you still be pushing on? No, you'll be driving your Cadillac to the golf club; only we nurses will be here, holding the bag. Are you going to provide the emotional support to us? We spend most our time here in the ICU providing high-level technical support to critically ill kids. Most of them are successes. We can deal with the few failures knowing that we've done our best. Tom's different; he won't get better. You know that. He'll just go from problem to problem. I can't take that forever."

"Barbara's right," states Jim. "The nurses will need support. But Rosa's going to need even more. How long do you think hope will sustain her? How long do you think she'll keep coming in every day? Soon it will be twice a week, then even less. What do you think that will do to her level of guilt? She's going to need a lot of support, maybe even a psychiatrist. Will the hospital pay for that? How long do you think the hospital will continue to foot Tom's bill?"

* * *

What are a physician's obligations to his patient? How are these obligations acquired? Do physicians acquire them by taking the Hippocratic oath? By virtue of an explicit promise to patients? Or in some other way? Explain how these commitments mandate the treatment you are providing for Tom. Are there any changes in Tom's condition that would lead you to change the level of medical care you feel should be provided?

What are Tom's rights? Does Tom have a right to this treatment because he is a human being, because he is a member of this society, or because of some explicit commitment that has been made to him? Does the fact that his survival occurred because of experimental surgery affect your commitment?

Professor Bradstreet's Argument: Calculating Social Benefit

"There's another way of looking at this," says Professor Bradstreet. "Our medical care system is in a mess. In the past 20 years our cost of medical care has gone from taking 5 percent of the gross national product to taking more than 10 percent. The recent federal changes in payment such as DRGs and cuts in funding are only the first attempts of the government to take control. It's going to get worse. If the medical care system does not do something to control costs and distribute those costs and care rationally, the bureaucrats will. And they don't understand the problems, only the bottom line.

"You know, it's peculiar, but no one wants to make decisions about individuals. We don't question the $100,000 for a heart transplant or the costs of kidney dialysis and transplantation—perhaps because we might need them one day. We spend unbelievable amounts on those small prematures, but darn little to prevent prematurity. You can't get funds for the public health measures that provide maximum benefit to large segments of the population, but it is there for the dramatic case. Look at all the money we spend on machines for the infant intensive care unit, and all the money spent on the cerebral palsy and retardation that result. Would some of that be better spent on prenatal clinics that might prevent babies from needing the intensive care? Granted, there is not enough money for everything, but shouldn't we allocate it for general social benefit, not just for individual benefit?

"Tom's case is a good example. Look at the past and future monetary expenditures, all because we thought we might be able to save one small child. The hospital could have spread the money to help lots of kids, or it could have started a clinic down the block that would have given health care, maybe even psychological care and educational help, to hundreds of inner-city kids. Which choice provides the most benefit? The problem is we don't like to make these decisions."

"You know, Bradstreet, that's a very interesting argument." Dr. Martin is a health care economist in the School of Public Health. "If you follow your social benefit arguments, Tom has some social benefit for himself; I'm not sure I can quantify it. He has some for his mother; at least that's her perception. Some little bit for society, since caring for the handicapped gives all of us some satisfaction. But there's a major debit for the individuals of society because, as you point out, we could use that money to help many more children who would be better contributors to society. At least if we set up prenatal clinics we could prevent more drains on society from cerebral palsy and mental retardation. I could easily see those utilitarian calculations coming out against Tom and for society. What then? What would you do? You could stop the dialysis, or whatever, to stop Tom's drain on society. But how would you assure that the funds saved went to society's benefit? In Tom's case it might be easier, since the money being spent is hospital money and you could make a deal with the hospital that you would turn off Tom if they promised to put the money in escrow to start the clinic next year, or something similar.

"What about all the other Toms out there across the country? Do you believe that the state legislature and the federal government would ever make a deal like that? Do you even think they would pass a law, saying 'no more heart transplants,' or 'no kidney transplants for persons over 60—they're not cost effective.'? Do you think they could decide 'no intensive care for infants less than 1½ pounds'? That would be political suicide. Congress can't even decide between B-1 bombers and ICBMs.

"Even if they did decide to limit health care, do you think that money would be allocated to prevention? To the greatest health care good for the greatest number? To education? I bet it would go for more cruise missiles, or a decrease in the national debt, perhaps a $3 rebate on your income tax. I don't believe that you can get where we may all want to go. Great idea, but it won't work!"

"It's very difficult to actually carry out the kind of social planning you advocate, Bradstreet," states the hospital chaplain. "It goes against the grain of our political system. The strength of our political system is its basis in individual freedom and diversity. You're talking about forcing people to do things, or preventing them from doing them. What about respect for the individual? That's been a key element in our political thinking.

"Was operating on Tom such a bad idea? Granted, it has had bad results, but we didn't know that this would be the outcome when the decision was made. Perhaps they've learned something and the next case will do better. You know, when they started open heart operations in the 1950s, the mortality was 80 percent, but the technique was finally perfected and now we're doing transplants. The same is true of prematures. Twenty years ago you would have cut off care at 3 to 4 pounds; now care and survival has been improved and you're proposing 1½ pounds as the cutoff. We wouldn't have made that progress if we stopped intensive care in the 1950s.

"But I have an even bigger problem. I'm not sure I trust the government to do social planning. They screw up frequently enough to be sure that they would decide on the wrong plan. They've done it before—look at B-1 bombers—and then they persist with the plan just because they made a decision. I'd rather foster diversity, try many different things, just allocate the money saved to health care and let a number of different programs flourish, given a certain amount of money."

Mr. Bergdorff of the hospital's board of trustees has slipped into the meeting. "You people are proposing a lot of fancy things," he says, "but I doubt you will establish federal policy in this committee. At least not today. You've forgotten that our problem is Tom and what this hospital should do about him. The hospital's job is to care for sick people, not to assess the value of these individuals to society. Some health care systems do ration health care, but those are societal decisions, not ones for this hospital or this committee to make. Until society changes its rules, we must honor our commitments."

* * *

Before you go on, think about where you stand on the arguments about individual and social benefits. Which should have primacy? What is the moral basis for choosing one over the other? How do you weigh the rights of the individual and your commitments to him against the rights of society and your obligation to it? How do you value diversity and freedom of choice against government policy?

If your arguments come out in favor of society, what would you do about Tom? What would that accomplish for society? What would that decision do to you and your role as a physician?

Jim and Barbara:
Parental Rights or Individual Benefits

Jim's argument is very persuasive. "In our society," he says, "parents have the right to decide how their children are to be treated. This right, of course, is not absolute. We do not allow parents to abuse their children or to fail to provide education or routine medical care. But within these boundaries, parents have tremendous latitude to decide. I've spoken to Tom's mother many times, most recently yesterday. She understands that Tom is way behind intellectually. She understands that it's unlikely that we'll ever be able to get him off the respirator and that he won't be a candidate for a kidney transplant. She understands that he's likely to be in the ICU for a long time, if not forever, and that this social deprivation is playing some role in his intellectual delay.

"But when I went over this again yesterday, she caught my drift that maybe it was time to cut back on support and let Tom die. She really lashed out; she was furious. She said something to the effect that it was great when those obstetrical doctors talked her into special surgery on Tom. They said everything would be fine. It was a terrific new idea. When Tom was born prematurely, they told her that he was lucky to be in a place with all the right machines and all the smart, dedicated doctors and nurses to help. She asked what's happened. Are they getting tired of Tom? Are all their new ideas not working? Now they want to dump him? She said that she was his mother and didn't abandon family when things get tough. She stuck with them. She emphasized that none of the things we are doing for Tom were heroic when we started doing them and she didn't see what made them special now. They were no more than what was being done for some of the other kids in the unit. At that point, she slammed down the phone.

"So I guess that settles it, at least for a long time. Tom's mother wants to stick with maximum therapy. From her perspective, I guess it makes a lot of sense. Of course, Father Rogers and I will work to bring her around to a more realistic perspective on Tom. But it sounds like that may take a while. It is her right to make the decision. She comes to visit all the time. If and when Tom ever gets out of here, no matter what condition he's in, she'll have to take care of him. Meanwhile, there is nothing to do but continue as we've been doing."

"I'm not convinced of that," said Barbara, Tom's principal nurse. "It will take a long time to bring Tom's mother around; you're right about that. But I don't see why that's necessary. Going back to what I said earlier, it's our responsibility to decide what's best for Tom. Once we figure out what's best, we have to sell it to whoever makes the decision.

"Now it's plain to me that we should stop supporting Tom, remove him from the respirator, and let him die. All we are doing now is causing him pain, misery, and suffering. It is fair to say that Tom has no real interest in staying alive. No reasonable person would want to live an entire life with tubes sticking out all over him. We have to act on Tom's best interests, and that means withdrawing support.

"But I don't think we should do this on our own. We should tell Tom's mother that if she won't agree, we will go to court and temporarily remove Tom from her custody. We will get the court to appoint a guardian to make a decision in Tom's interest, and then we will withdraw support. We need to be understanding but firm with her. We must remember, however, that Tom is our patient and that we must do what's best for him."

Father Rogers intervened at this point. "I find myself in between your position and Jim's. I agree that Tom's condition is hopeless, but I also think that Tom's mother should make the decision, and I don't like the idea of going to court. I propose that we set things up so that Tom's mother comes around quickly to allowing us to disconnect Tom's support systems. I do not share Jim's willingness to let Tom suffer while we wait for Rosa to see things reasonably.

"We need to take a two-pronged approach to this problem. First, psychologically, we need to relieve Rosa of any guilt she might feel. She always talks as though cutting off support is abandoning Tom. Instead of presenting it as her decision, we've got to present it as ours and just ask her to go along. It's unfair to ask her to bear that burden of guilt. How can she say she's abandoning her son?

"Second, we have to show her just how much discomfort our procedures cause Tom. We have to get her to watch when somebody's putting down a nasogastric tube. And we have to show her how blue Tom gets when we disconnect the respirator to suction him. We have to get her to look at some of the junk we take out of his lungs:

"We can't just let Tom's mother float along waiting for her to make up her own mind. We have to help her make the right decision.

"Jim, my son, you don't think we're being paternalistic, do you?"

* * *

If you want to decide what is best for Tom, how do you calculate his best interest? Obviously, Rosa, Jim, Barbara, and Father Rogers each have somewhat different views of his best interests and how to achieve them. Who should decide? What would you do? Do you wish to take Jim's go-slow approach, or do you prefer Father Rogers' more paternalistic, aggressive approach? Do you think Barbara is right and that you should get a court to take Tom from his mother's custody so that his best interests will be served?

Should this case be decided on the basis of Tom's best interest, or on choosing the right person to decide? Or should it follow Bernie's argument and continue treatment because that is what physicians do best?

What are Tom's best interests? To die or to continue indefinitely in his present state? Should his interests be considered narrowly or broadly; that is, should family and social interests be factored in, or should one consider only what is best for Tom as an individual? Reconsider Professor Bradstreet's arguments. If you look at Tom only as an individual, is Barbara right in thinking that he is better off dead? How does one know whether continued life is in one's interests?

If Tom's interests are not clear, does the issue come down to who has the right to decide? Is that right based on expertise or on socially accepted roles? If Tom's mother has the right to decide, is her right based on knowledge of what is best for Tom or on her role as Tom's mother? If the right to decide is based on expertise, who is the expert and how does that expert decide what is best? If it is based on social roles or position, who should make the decision, and what is the moral warrant for these social roles?

Prepare a memo for the staff explaining and justifying your decision. Carefully develop the moral theory on which your decision is based. If there are rights involved, exactly what are they, who has them, where do they come from, and what are their limits? If the issue is Tom's interests, how are they determined, and on what moral theory are they based?

You have now heard all the arguments and thought about the moral basis behind them. What will you do about Tom? Why will you do it?

Chapter 6

Marti Revisited

"Since we did so well with discussions about Tom last week," you say, "shall we try to make some plans for Marti? Let me fill Mrs. Dow in about Marti. Mrs. Dow represents the State Crippled Children's Agency.

"Marti, as most of you know, is a C2 spinal cord transection caused by an automobile accident. She is totally and permanently paralyzed from the neck down and can't even breathe for herself. Her mind is intact; indeed, she was one of the top students in her class, intellectually and athletically. It's very sad. She says she wants to be dead. It's been more than three months since the accident, so nothing physical is likely to change.

"If we were to listen to Marti, we would give her a tranquilizer and pull the plug on her respirator immediately. She has been talking about this for at least two weeks. What do your people in psychiatry think, Dr. Walsh?"

"Marti is a very depressed young lady. Considering her condition, of course, that is not at all surprising. It's only three months since her accident. Depression is an expected and normal stage in the process of recovery. At this point it is outrageous to think of Marti's making any decision at all about her care, much less her life.

"Marti has stopped denying some of her injury and has started the painful process of learning to live with it. Our job is to help her work through this adjustment."

"How long do you think it will take her to get over her depression?" you ask.

"I don't think she will ever *completely* recover," replies Dr. Walsh candidly. "Compared with those born with physical handicaps, people who acquire them by injury are much less likely to adapt fully to their condition. Something has been taken away from them; they've been robbed, so to speak. They never completely get over it.

57

"Marti, therefore, will probably need help with recurrent depression for a long time. If, from time to time, she expresses suicidal wishes, we will take that as evidence of depression and deal with it appropriately. It would also be evidence of our failure in rehabilitation; we would just have to try harder to help her accommodate."

"Sounds like a catch 22," comments Barbara. "If you want to die, you're crazy, but if you're crazy, you aren't competent to make the decision to die."

"There may be some truth to that, Barbara," Dr. Walsh continues, "but I think the responsibility of medicine is to help people live their lives and adapt to their circumstances. Many quadriplegics lead adequate, even satisfying, lives. Depression is a treatable condition and, like other illnesses, it is our job to treat it. The issue is not just suicide. If she is unhappy, she needs our help. She may need our help for a long time."

"As we discussed last week when we were talking about Tom's case," Professor Bradstreet grumbled, "this is a question about what is best for society, not just for Marti. Her care is going to cost society millions of dollars over her lifetime. She will never make any contribution. But, unlike Tom, we know what she wants—to die. Social utility theory would suggest that we should let her die, and we should use the money saved to educate the children down the street.

"This is certainly not the right body to make these decisions. Unfortunately, society does not allow anyone to make socially responsible decisions in such a situation as this."

"Excuse me, but I am very uncomfortable with even raising these issues of social utility," says Ms. Dow, angrily twisting her wheelchair back and forth at the table. "The policy of the Crippled Children's Service is to do anything and everything we can to rehabilitate these children. Allocating our contribution on the basis of expected social contribution is immoral, undemocratic, and probably illegal."

"Allocation of resources is just not the issue at all," began Sara, Marti's principal nurse. "Our society is not based on how it spends its money, but on its respect for individuals and their decisions. That is what democracy is all about. In all the material on medical ethics I've been reading in the nursing journals, respecting the autonomy of the individual is the key to moral decision making. I have to disagree with Dr. Walsh because he is advocating paternalism. He won't, in effect, let Marti make a decision that he doesn't consider rational, healthy, and beneficial. Professor Bradstreet is paternalistic, too. His, of course, is 'Big Brother' paternalism. Don't all of us have the right to make decisions about how we will be cared for while alive, or the right to end that life if we choose?

"Marti is 12 years old, and she is fairly mature. I agree with Dr. Walsh that Marti is depressed right now and that she should not make any immediate decisions. We will have to wait, perhaps even a year or more, before we see if she can adjust to her quadriplegia. But then her life should be her own decision."

Barbara, Tom's nurse, supports Sara. "In Tom's case I think we are substituting our judgment for his own—a judgment that, as an infant, he obviously cannot make. That is not the case here. I agree with Sara that this is Marti's decision."

"Well, that's not so clear to me," said Dr. Graeme, one of the senior pediatricians. "How many of you are parents? How many parents would let their 12-year-olds make decisions like this? This patient autonomy business is fine for mature adults, but we're dealing with a child whose parents closely supervise everything she does—the television shows she watches, the movies she goes to, the friends she has over. They are pretty careful about what she does. Now you're going to let this child make an irrevocable decision about her own death? That's crazy! Marti has a perfectly normal 12-year-old intellect and 12-year-old emotions, which is why she is utterly incapable of making this decision. I know that I'm speaking as a mother," Dr. Graeme continued, "but that experience should count for something.

"Furthermore, she has an intact and loving family. They're very committed to caring for her. We should do nothing at all to separate her from that care. It's not our business to push her toward autonomy. Her family has reasonable ideas about Marti's life. These people want to provide good, customary medicine. They are not fanatics who are turning away from standard care. The burden of proof has to rest on those who would reject standard care, and there is no way that a 12-year-old can shoulder that burden.

"I realize, of course, that the day will come when Marti will make her own decisions. But that day is many years away; it is not our concern now, or any time soon."

"I'm sorry to have to disagree with you, Dr. Graeme," Sara begins. "We start from the same point but end up very differently.

"Marti is a perfectly normal 12-year-old, and I know that life is asking a lot of her. It's all very unfair, of course, but that's how it is; it's her decision.

"My position is very simple, but let me read a passage from my medical ethics text quoting an old court decision:

> No right is held more sacred, or is more carefully guarded by the common law, than the right of every individual to the possession and control of his own person, free from all restraint or interference by others, unless by clear and unquestionable authority of law.
>
> *Union Pacific Railway Company* v. *Botsford* (1891)

59

"The right to self-determination has a basis in law, and a moral basis in personal autonomy. Lots of philosophers talk about it; it's part of our constitution and part of our whole society.

"Now I have to admit that it isn't clear exactly how this applies to Marti. It's tough when teenagers have to make decisions like this. And I don't suppose anyone is ever mature enough. I know I would be terrified; I wouldn't have the guts to tell them to pull the plug on me.

"The only thing that counts is that Marti has the right to decide her own fate. It's reasonable to stall for a little bit, at least until she gets over the initial shock. But everything turns on what she decides. It's her life."

"It may be her life, but it's our respirator," puts in Bernie. "She can do anything she wants, or can get someone else to do it, but not while she's in our care. It's fine with me if we get her out of here and if she persuades somebody in a nursing home or even her parents to pull the plug for her. But while she's our patient, she gives up some of her autonomy.

"Remember the case of the woman in California who got herself admitted to a hospital and then didn't want them to feed her with a nasogastric tube? The hospital got a court to support its argument that it could determine appropriate medical care as long as the woman was its patient.

"If Marti wants to control her medical care, she'll have to get out of here."

"You bastard," sputtered Barbara, "that's mean. Aren't we here to serve our patients? Aren't we all in health care to help people? If that little girl pleaded with you to do something for her, you wouldn't do it? What kind of patient service is that? None at all! Just because she's in a hospital you impose limits on her autonomy, boundaries on what she can decide. What gives you the right to do that? Our job is to take care of patients, to put their needs first. Does she have to sign out against medical advice to get the care she needs? She didn't even come here voluntarily; the ambulance brought her."

"Hold on just a second," interrupted Dr. Graeme. "Neither of you are seeing the whole picture. I agree with Barbara and Sara that this is a question of *who* should decide. But how can you take a 12-year-old out of the context of her family? No 12-year-old, indeed very few of us, has the kind of individual autonomy that you two are talking about. Aren't our husbands, wives, children, and parents involved in any important decisions we make, especially life or death decisions?

"I also agree just a little with Bernie. We have to have a bias for treatment. Only if both Marti and her family were firm in their decision and held to it for a good period of time would I agree to take her off the respirator. Under those circumstances, I would do it; I would not pass the buck to a nursing home or anybody else."

I hate to interfere in this very serious discussion," says Mr. Bergdorf, the hospital trustee, "but when you are making this decision, I don't think you should let cost enter into it. If there are problems paying for Marti's care, I'm sure the trustees' fund will help out. We are building an extended care wing on the hospital, and Marti could even be a help to us in fund raising."

* * *

What do you think of Dr. Walsh's catch 22? Does a person have a right to commit suicide, or is that wish a sign of depression and therefore of emotional incompetence requiring treatment? Is suicide ever rational?

Would you agree with Dr. Graeme that this is far too important a decision to leave a 12-year-old? At what age could someone make such a decision? Is it ever reasonable to leave the decision solely to the individual, without involvement of family and friends?

If you believe in autonomy, how do you rebut these arguments? Is anyone ever totally autonomous? Does admission to the hospital limit a patient's autonomy? Why? Why do we make patients sign out against medical advice instead of just saying good-bye?

Does Mr. Bergdorf's offer of financial assistance and his eagerness to use Marti's condition for fund raising alter the arguments?

Having considered these arguments, what would be your plan for Marti? On what basis would you make it, and how would you morally defend it?

Chapter 7

Mr. Edgar Jones

"Molly," you call out as you walk into the waiting room outside the operating suite. Molly, sitting in the far corner of the room and waiting for her husband to come out of surgery, looks up from her crossword puzzle. "We have to talk. Let's go to the conference room across the hall." Molly is in her middle 50s, a former nurse, and now head of the Women's Auxiliary here at Community Hospital. You have been close friends with Molly and Edgar Jones for years. You and Edgar are part of the same Wednesday golf foursome. This is not going to be an easy discussion.

Edgar Jones is a 55-year-old chemical engineer. You are a general surgeon at Community. Edgar is a healthy specimen, admitted now for removal of a gallstone. You have been the Jones' surgeon before, luckily being there for Edgar's emergency appendectomy and referring Molly elsewhere for a consultation before ultimately doing a lumpectomy when most of the other surgeons in the area would have done a radical mastectomy.

Everything seemed to be going well in the operating room when you noticed that Edgar's tissues were turning blue. Checking with the anesthesiologist, a new man you had not worked with often, you found that something was wrong. The anesthesiologist worked rapidly with his machines, but Edgar's blood pressure had dropped precipitously, and a quick listen with the stethescope revealed a cardiac arrest. The anesthesiologist administered stimulants while you ordered and used the defibrillator. You had no idea of the cause of the problem. Did the anesthesia tube dislodge? Although it seemed like an eternity, it took perhaps four or five minutes, maybe more, to get Edgar's heart going again. Had there been enough oxygen to maintain the brain during that time? Would Edgar recover? Would he be impaired? If so, how great would the damage be? The outcome is not at all clear at this point. The session with Molly is going to be very painful.

Mr. Edgar Jones

"What's the matter?" asks Molly as you walk into the waiting room. "Is Edgar okay? Did you find a growth or something? Didn't things go well?"

From the look on your face it is clear that there has been trouble.

"Sit down, Molly," you say, "we've got a real problem. I am not entirely sure that I know what happened, but there must have been a problem with the anesthesia. Edgar's heart arrested on the table. We got it going again. As you know, the brain can only stand three or four minutes without oxygen, and we can't be exactly sure how much brain damage occurred. It could be considerable. For anyone else, we would just go ahead, sew up, and send the patient to the intensive care unit. But you and I have been close enough so that I think you should be part of what could be a very crucial decision.

"I can't help but remember all the discussions that we've had about medical technology and the foolishness of keeping patients going when there's nothing good to come of it. In the last few minutes I've been thinking about Edgar's vehement statements that he'd never want to just cling to life, hooked to a machine. He hates the idea of being dependent or a burden. Edgar is much too vigorous and self-sufficient for that. Well, everything Edgar fears is a real possibility now.

"It's possible, of course, that Edgar's brain and heart suffered such a severe insult that he won't make it no matter what we do. But I don't think the cardiac arrest lasted that long. It's also possible, on the other side, that we caught all this in time and that Edgar will come out with little or no damage. That's not likely either. I'm afraid the biggest chance is for something in between, that Edgar's brain will be impaired, perhaps even severely impaired. If it is severely impaired, he might not be able to talk, to care for himself, or even to think. He could survive for weeks, even years, in such a state. I just don't know."

There is a terrible pause as Molly sobs quietly.

"Marcus, isn't there any hope?" she asks. "Can't you do anything? I love him so much, but I don't want him to suffer. Why did this have to happen? He is such a good man and a good husband. Isn't there any hope?"

You put your arm around Molly's shoulder. "There is hope, Molly, but not very much, and we could pay a tremendous price for it. If we bring him to the ICU and put him on a respirator, there's a very good chance that he'll survive, but there's also a great risk he'll be substantially impaired. On the other hand, if we disconnect him now, there is no real hope of his survival."

* * *

63

What should you do now? This is the optimal time to avoid the risk of prolonged impairment for Edgar. If you disconnect the anesthesia machine he will certainly die. There will be no chance of survival with impairment. There will also be no chance of survival without impairment.

If there was a 10-percent chance of good recovery, would you deny Edgar that chance? How about a 5-percent chance? A 2-percent chance? Does the percentage chance make a difference, since the ultimate outcome will be all or none?

This option of turning off the anesthesia machine, while theoretically possible, is not realistic. It is not acceptable practice to turn off the machine in the operating room while there is even a small chance of a good recovery. Should this standard of good practice be changed?

Edgar Goes to the ICU

You return to the operating room as the residents are finishing up. Edgar seems to be stable, but there is no way of knowing how much damage has been done. The anesthesia has been allowed to wear off, but Edgar is not yet breathing on his own and continues to require a respirator. Despite your concern for him and his wife, you follow the standard procedure and send Edgar to intensive care.

After watching the stretcher disappear down the hall, you return to the conference room to talk with Molly.

"I thought this through as best I could, Molly, and we had a quick discussion in the operating room. As much as I would like to be sure that Edgar won't suffer, we *have* to keep him in the ICU and see what happens. We'll do everything we can to support him now. Tomorrow we'll do an electroencephalogram (EEG), a test of his brainwaves. That may give us some clues about his recovery, but the clinical signs are more important. Most people who are going to recover will show a dramatic response in two or three days. If Edgar is not doing well and the EEG shows extensive damage, we can consider turning off the respirator.

"You'll be able to see Edgar in the ICU in about half an hour. Don't be frightened by all the equipment around his bed: the respirator, cardiac monitors, IV lines, and catheters. They're all part of standard care in that unit. There is nothing to do now but hope and pray."

*　　*　　*

Do you feel comfortable with this decision? Have you made this decision because you thought it best or because you "had no choice?" Did you lack choice because you feared the legal consequences of letting Edgar die on the operating table, because you think that physicians must always follow standard medical practice, or because you believe that you are required to do everything reasonable for a patient as long as there is *any* chance for his recovery?

Does Mr. Jones have the right to refuse medical treatment? If so, how could he exercise this right? Is there any way he could have done so before the surgery? Considering the possibility that he will recover, would a "living will" or equivalent document have been helpful?

Is there a moral basis for the decision you have made, or is your decision based entirely on legal grounds or on standard medical practice? Do you have an obligation as a treating surgeon to continue treatment when there is *any* reasonable chance of a good recovery? How do you define reasonable? After thinking carefully about these questions, continue reading the case.

Three Days Later

It is now three long days since the operation. Edgar Jones remains on a respirator; he is not able to breathe on his own. His blood pressure and heart rate are normal. He responds only to intense pain, and then only in minimal fashion. He is deeply comatose. Yesterday's EEG has been read, and a note from the neurologist says that it shows evidence of severe brain dysfunction. Because there is some brain activity, however, Edgar is not brain dead. He has not shown the dramatic response for which you and Molly were hoping.

You spot Molly as you leave the ICU. She looks fatigued and depressed. You have been talking to her once or twice a day, trying to keep up her hope. Now it is time to face it. You take her to the ICU conference room.

"Molly," you begin, "things look very bad. Edgar shows no sign of waking up. I'm afraid our worst fears are coming true. It's now clear that he has suffered severe and permanent brain injury. Patients who are going to make a good recovery virtually all show some positive response by now. Edgar is hardly responsive at all. We can see from the EEG that he suffered severe damage, and the finding confirms our clinical exam. On the other hand, Edgar is not dead; he does not meet the established criteria for brain death. I don't know how long he could go on like this, but with good nursing care and the respirator, it could be a long time: weeks, months, or even years. This is the state he was most afraid of and did not want. All we're doing now with our high-technology medicine is prolonging his dying. And he would enjoy no reasonable life in the meantime.

"It may be time for us to stop, time to turn off the respirator. Since Edgar requires the machine to breathe, stopping it would be a merciful way of allowing him to die. Many people say that this is not killing him, but merely removing the technology that is artificially preserving his life. While some patients in Edgar's condition live on in a vegetative state, it's exceedingly unlikely that he would return to anything like normal human function. What do you think we should do?"

"Marcus, I don't know," replies Molly. "I love him so much that even just sitting by his bedside is a great comfort to me. I can't bear to think of life without him. But I know how he felt about this. He wouldn't want to be kept alive in this state. He wouldn't want to be a burden—but I don't find him a burden. Do what you think best. You're our close friend, not just our doctor."

* * *

Now you must make a decision. At this point, postponement is as much a decision as any other. Think very carefully, because your decision may be irrevocable.

If you decide to leave Edgar on the respirator and review the situation in two weeks, turn to "Edgar Continues on the Respirator" (p. 71).

If you decide to turn off the respirator, consider the justification for your decision. Is it justified by Edgar's wishes, by Molly's acquiescence, by what is best for Edgar, or by some combination of these three? Would you still disconnect the respirator if one of these factors were missing? If two were missing?

After thinking about these factors, if you still want to turn off the respirator, flip a coin to find what happens. If it comes up heads, continue with the following section. If it comes up tails, see "Tails" on p. 68.

Heads: You Plan to Turn Off the Respirator

"Molly," you say, "I think we've done all we can. Edgar would want us to stop. Do you want to say good-bye before I turn off the machine?"

You stand with your arm around Molly's shoulder while she says her tearful good-byes. After a parting kiss to Edgar, Molly leaves the room.

Mr. Edgar Jones

Elenore, the head nurse in the ICU, comes over. "What's happening, Doctor?"

"Elenore," you begin "we've reached the end of the road. It's time to turn off the respirator. Molly and I have had a long talk. It's what Mr. Jones would want, and it's what we think is best. What do you think?"

"That's what I would want if it were me," she replies, "but he's not brain dead, so we can't do it. You're too valuable to this hospital and to your patients to take the risk of going against established procedures. Please, go to the Ethics Committee. If they say it's okay, you won't have any problems. We don't want that district attorney coming around here again."

"You know, Elenore, it's not like it used to be, when we doctors could do what was best for our patients. All these rules and regulations interfere with the practice of good medicine. But you're right, I'll talk to the committee first. I guess I'd better call Molly, too."

As you stop by the doctor's lounge to sign out of the hospital, you run into Dr. Baldwin, chairman of the Ethics Committee.

"Bill," you smile, "I'm glad to see you. I was going to call you this afternoon about your committee. I guess I need their approval. You know about what happened to Edgar Jones the other day. Well, he's still in the ICU and not responding at all. I think it's time to quit, to turn off the respirator. Elenore, the head nurse up there, says that, since he's not brain dead, I better run it by your committee. What do you think?"

"How long has it been since the cardiac arrest?" asks Bill.

"Three days."

"His EEG, is it flat? Has he got brainstem responses?"

"The EEG's bad, but not flat. But there's not much brainstem function."

"Then he's not officially brain dead, and it's too early to be sure that he's chronically and irreversibly comatose. I'd be happy to present it to the committee, but I know what they're going to say. Sorry, Marcus, but there's no easy way out. If he gets pneumonia and you don't recognize and treat it, if he gets phlebitis and a pulmonary embolus, or if he has a heart attack, then he'll be lucky. You certainly should write a no-code order, but you can't do anything active like pulling the plug."

"Pulling the plug isn't active, Bill. He'd die from not breathing due to the brain damage. What's the difference between that and dying of pneumonia or something else that I carefully don't treat?"

"Marcus, we're in foolish times. The Committee doesn't make the rules; we just try to help keep physicians out of trouble. Others worry about the subtle distinction between active and passive. Sorry."

Turn to "The Respirator Continues" (p. 68).

Tails: The Respirator Is Turned Off

Molly comes to be with Edgar when he dies. She holds his hand while you turn off the respirator. As you both stand there, Edgar Jones does not breathe. He turns a little blue, and his heart rate drops to seventy, then to sixty. After three minutes it goes to fifty, then to forty. He takes a big gasp, and his heartbeat increases to fifty-five. Thirty seconds later he takes another gasp, followed by several more. Then he begins to breathe on his own. Damn! His heart rate returns to normal and his breathing becomes regular. You predicted that it was only your machine that was keeping him alive, but you were wrong.

You and Molly both walk out of the ICU and speechlessly enter a conference room. You sit down together, but neither says anything for a long time.

"I just don't know what to do, Molly. I don't know what to say. We'll just see how it goes for the next week or so."

Then you help the sobbing woman to her car.

Turn to "Two Weeks Later," page 69.

The Respirator Continues

It's now more than a week since the surgery, and Edgar continues to rest comfortably in the ICU. He remains on the respirator and is fed intravenously. He still doesn't breathe on his own and remains deeply comatose. The EEG shows a bit of abnormal activity.

Molly sits down in your office for another of what have become increasingly awful discussions.

"Molly," you begin, "last night I spoke again with Bill Baldwin, chairman of the Ethics Committee, and he agrees that now we can turn off the respirator. Although Edgar isn't brain dead, he's more like Karen Ann Quinlan—irreversibly comatose. Bill thinks we'd be legally and morally in the clear. Is that okay with you?"

"Marcus, we should have done it in the operating room. It's been a terrible week. I don't know if he's suffered as much as I have; perhaps he can't feel anything, but if he knew, he would be suffering. Yes, it's time for him to be relieved of all this."

Mr. Edgar Jones

Molly comes into the ICU to be with Edgar when he dies. She holds his hand while you turn off the respirator. As you stand there, Edgar does not breathe. He turns a little blue, and his heart rate drops to seventy, then to sixty. After three minutes it goes to fifty, then to forty. He takes a big gasp, and his heartbeat increases to fifty-five. Thirty seconds later he takes another gasp, followed by several more. Then he begins to breathe on his own. Damn! His heart rate returns to normal and his breathing becomes regular. You predicted that it was only your machinery that was keeping him alive, but you were wrong.

You and Molly walk out of the ICU together and speechlessly enter a conference room. You both sit down, but neither says anything for a long time.

"I just don't know what to do, Molly. I don't know what to say. We'll just see how it goes."

Then you help the sobbing woman to her car.

Two Weeks Later

It's now two weeks since surgery, and you call Molly. "Molly," you say, "I've been thinking, and about the only option left to us is to discontinue the feeding tube. If we continue as we've been going, Edgar could linger forever, unless he's lucky enough to get some fatal complications. We will have to move him to a nursing home so that your insurance will last longer. If we stop the feeding tube, we'll be depriving him of fluids and nutrition. It might take a week or so for him to die if we do that but, since he's comatose, there shouldn't be any pain or suffering.

"I've been doing a bit of research," you continue. "There was a patient just like Edgar, where the doctors stopped feeding him with his wife's agreement. He died and the district attorney wanted to prosecute them for murder. The appeals court [*Barber* v. *L.A. County Superior Court;* California Court of Appeals] found that since feeding him wasn't going to improve his condition, the physicians weren't under a legal obligation to continue. Thus, they couldn't be found criminally negligent.

"There's also a different case in New Jersey, the Claire Conroy case, [*In the Matter of Claire C. Conroy,* Supreme Court of New Jersey, 1983] which applied different standards but came to the same conclusion. Although the medical situation was somewhat different because Miss Conroy was already dying, the court outlined three general tests for withdrawing life support equipment: subjective, limited objective, and objective.

69

The court ruled that medical treatment could be withdrawn if any one of these three tests were satisfied.

"The court called the first test 'subjective' because it preserves the rights of individual subjects to make decisions about their own care: 'The goal of decision making for incompetent patients should be to determine and effectuate, insofar as possible, the decision that the patient would have made if competent.'

"You and I both know Edgar's wishes about this situation; unfortunately, we don't have a living will or any other written documentation. Although the Conroy court was very cautious and required extensive verification of the patient's wishes, I feel very comfortable that this would be Edgar's decision.

"The two versions of the objective are not as helpful in our situation. These tests require that the patient is in 'recurring, unavoidable, and severe pain' or that continued treatment of the patient be 'inhumane.' Since Edgar is comatose, he doesn't have pain, and the term 'inhumane' is too vague.

"In many ways, Edgar is like Karen Quinlan. He is chronically and irreversibly comatose and, like Karen, he said he didn't want to be maintained on machines. The courts gave guardianship to Karen's parents to make the decision about the respirator. In the Conroy case the court said that feeding tubes are technology just like a respirator. I have the statement here; let me read it to you."

> However, artificial feedings such as nasogastric tubes, gastrostomies, and intravenous infusion are . . . medical procedures with inherent risks and possible side effects, instituted by skilled health-care providers to compensate for impaired physical functioning. Analytically, artificial feeding by means of a nasogastric tube or intravenous infusion can been seen as equivalent to artificial breathing by means of a respirator.

"Following their reasoning, I think we could stop feeding Edgar. What's your opinion?"

"Well," Molly says, "I don't know about *analytically* and all those things lawyers worry about, but it just doesn't feel the same to take the food and water away from him. Edgar always so enjoyed the meals I cooked; he was always a steak and potatoes man. I mean, respirators are funny little machines with tubes hanging all over them. But I've been in nursing; a nasogastric tube is the most ordinary thing in the world. How can we take that away from him? Even though he can't feel it, how can we take away his nourishment? How can we let him die of thirst?

"I know you've always done what you thought best and I've always thought you've done what is best for Edgar. I know that it's just a wife's emotion, but taking away his water just doesn't *feel* right to me."

* * *

What will you say to Molly? *Is* taking away food and water provided by a nasogastric tube the same as taking away a respirator? Remember that taking away a respirator takes away the air we breathe. Is there a distinction between killing Edgar and letting him die? When you removed the respirator, he breathed on his own. But if you take away the nasogastric tube, he cannot eat on his own. Removing that tube will surely result in his death. Is that different from killing him? Can you make a distinction between killing him and stopping futile or "heroic" care, even though you recognize that he will die because you stopped therapy?

If stopping care is not different from killing him, why not do just that? Why should it take a week or more to let him die, inefficiently, perhaps even painfully, when that result could be achieved in minutes?

How should you go about making this decision? Molly is reluctant, but doubtless could be brought around. How hard should you work at persuading her? Does trying to persuade her mean that you are exerting undue pressure? Does it mean that she is less free to make a decision?

What ethical theories justify the decisions you have been making? Have you respected Edgar's rights? Molly's rights? Have you done your duty as a physician? Have you overdone it? Have you done what is best for Edgar? For Molly? For society as a whole?

Carefully consider these issues before you make a decision. If you decide not to remove the feeding tube , turn to "You Just Could Not Remove the Feeding Tube" (p. 73). If you decide to remove the tube, turn to the "Discussion" (p. 74).

Edgar Continues on the Respirator

You've decided to maintain Edgar on the respirator. Two weeks have passed since the surgery, and his vital signs remain stable. Edgar is now fed by a tube that goes through his nose. There is no improvement, but neither is he getting worse.

The total cost of Edgar's stay in the ICU is $1,500 per day. Insurance covers most of this, but Molly must pay 20 percent. In three weeks, however, Edgar will reach the limits of his policy, and the burden will be all on Molly.

You cannot transfer him to the ward because hospital policy forbids respirator-dependent patients outside the ICU. (The hospital had some very expensive experiences in court, and the rule is strictly enforced.) Indeed, standard medicine requires a tracheotomy at this point to keep Edgar on the respirator. This is a simple procedure to insert a breathing tube in his throat. Caring for a patient with a tracheotomy requires specially experienced nurses and therefore drastically limits the facilities outside the hospital that might care for Edgar.

If you elect to turn off the respirator now, turn back to "Tails: The Respirator Is Turned Off" (p. 68).

If you elect to continue the respirator, can you continue to face Molly? How will you help her to bear the psychological strain of seeing Edgar in a hopeless condition, dependent on the machines he hated? How will you help her with the financial burdens involved in Edgar's care? Would you advise her to sell the house to pay the bills?

Write a letter to Molly explaining why you have persisted in keeping Edgar on a respirator. In the letter, appeal specifically to the moral theory on which you based your decision. Would disconnecting Edgar violate his right to life? Would it be killing him? Is keeping Edgar on the machine required by your duty as a physician? How do your answers to these questions relate to the moral theory you are using?

Could there be a change in Edgar's situation that would lead you to disconnect him from the machine? Are you committed to keeping patients like Edgar going no matter what? Would you consider increasing the level of therapy? How, for example, will you treat the pneumonias he will eventually develop? Will you use whatever antibiotics it will take? Do you think that it is wrong to discontinue therapy once it is begun but acceptable not to begin new therapies? Use your moral theory to develop and justify this distinction.

After you have written this letter, turn to the "Discussion" on page 74.

You Just Could Not Remove
the Feeding Tube

You have decided to maintain Edgar on the feeding tube. Another several weeks have passed, and he remains stable. There is no improvement, but neither is he getting any worse.

The total cost of Edgar's stay in the ICU was $1500 per day. Now, on the hospital ward, it is $500 per day. Insurance covers most of this, but Molly must pay 20 percent. Soon, however, Edgar will reach the limits of his policy and the burden will be all on Molly.

Now you must transfer Edgar to a nursing home where the care will be cheaper and he will not occupy a bed needed for acute patients. Can you continue to face Molly? How will you help her to bear the psychological strain of seeing Edgar in a hopeless medical condition, totally dependent on the type of care he hated? How will you help her with the financial burdens involved in Edgar's care? Would you advise her to sell the house to pay the bills?

Write a letter to Molly explaining why you have persisted in keeping Edgar on the tube feeding. In the letter, appeal specifically to the moral theory on which you based your decision. Would disconnecting Edgar violate his right to life? Would it be killing him? Is feeding Edgar required by your duty as a physician? Is it a benefit to him or to society?

Is there anything you will leave out of the letter? Are you going to discuss the legal ramifications of not feeding Edgar? Are you going to discuss the hospital's or your own financial interests in the case? How do your answers to these questions relate to the moral theory you are using?

Could there be a change in Edgar's situation that would lead you to discontinue feeding him? Are you committed to keeping patients like Edgar going no matter what else might happen, such as a heart attack? Would you consider increasing the level of therapy in that situation? How, for example, will you treat the pneumonias he will eventually develop? Will you use whatever antibiotics it will take? Do you think that it is wrong to discontinue a course of therapy once it is begun but acceptable not to begin new therapies? Use your moral theory to develop and justify this distinction.

After you have written this letter, turn to the "Discussion" on page 74.

Discussion

You have just gone through a common scenario for many patients with strokes, severe head injuries, cardiac arrests, or even surgical misadventures. This case is a composite of several situations, but it describes events that can and do happen.

If, at any later time, you decide to disconnect him from the respirator or discontinue his feeding line, it would have been better if you had done it sooner. Then you would have avoided the long time on the respirator, the suffering of the family and, most of all, you would have followed Edgar Jones' fervent wishes. But, in the operating room, was there any way to know whether he would recover? Without such knowledge, would not resuscitating him have been a wise decision? Only the subsequent hours, days, or weeks would reveal the severity of the brain damage and the degree of Edgar's recovery.

If Edgar had awakened, the decision to keep him on the respirator would have been best. And had Edgar died, or had he met all the standard criteria for brain death, there would have been no moral problem. But keeping him on a respirator entails the risk that he will remain neither brain dead nor alert. The longer you maintain care, the greater the chance that he will survive in some limbo state. The demands of good emergency decision making militates against insuring the best outcome for Edgar Jones.

There could be an alternative way of facing these problems in which it is possible to avoid the Hobson's choice between risking the loss of a salvageable patient and risking the survival of a patient in a persistent vegetative state. Better decisions could be made if there were more knowledge of the patient's condition and less of the pressure of an emergency. Consider the following revision of the beginning of this case.

You leave the operating room for a discussion with Molly. Taking her from the waiting room to a conference room, you explain the anesthetic mishap and tell her that you do not know what the consequences will be. You explain that the best course of action is to provide maximum care for Edgar: put him on a respirator, get an EEG, and see what happens over the next few days.

"Molly," you continue, "I think the chances of Edgar's making a full recovery are small, but we should give him every chance. Despite every-thing we do, he may not make it. But if he survives and is severely im-paired, I can assure you that he will not suffer either pain or the indig-nities of a severely damaged life. As Edgar, you, and I have discussed several times, he does not want to live that way. And he does not want to put you through the agony of his lingering in a chronic vegetative state.

"His wish to avoid this can be accomplished swiftly and painlessly by injection once it becomes obvious that he will not regain consciousness. The hospital has a Euthanasia Committee that understands these situa-tions. If we get to that point, the committee will review the case to insure that the family and the physicians are acting as the patient would have wanted. If we see clearly that Edgar is going to be severely impaired, we can ask the committee to go over the case carefully and talk with us, affording legal protection to all concerned.

"The existence of the committee makes the present decision easy. We can go all out for Edgar, giving him the best chance for a good recovery. Yet we also know that we have an escape if things do not go as we hope.

"Three or four days from now, or whenever the situation is clarified, and if things aren't going well, we'll call in the Euthanasia Committee. After consulting with them, we could turn off the respirator. If Edgar breathes at this point, we could give him an injection of potassium that would stop his heart and allow him to die swiftly and painlessly.

"We won't be forced to stand by helplessly, waiting for Edgar to get a pneumonia that we won't treat. Edgar and everyone else will be spared the agony of a lingering, perhaps painful, death. With an injection, he can have a good death—euthanasia. That's what the term means."

* * *

There are no euthanasia committees; the scenario presented here is im-possible under current law. Assume that a congressional committee is considering euthanasia legislation and write a letter to the committee voicing your opinion.

No matter what your ultimate position, consider the pragmatic advan-tages and disadvantages of any such proposal. It would offer patients in Edgar Jones' position the most vigorous possible therapy. What would be the effect of such legislation on patients or families who would reject a euthanasia option? What safeguards would be required for the operation of such a committee? Should anyone involved be able to reject euthana-sia: patient, physician, family? What should the committee do when a family is divided? How would one insure that such committees did not take advantage of the weak, the handicapped, and the defenseless? Should the committees use an adversarial system to prevent abuses?

Most important, take a position on the morality of euthanasia and rebut the arguments of your opponents. Appeal as explicitly as possible to moral theory in support of your view.

Euthanasia—a good death—will be one of the major ethical issues of the next decade. We are increasingly debating decisions about embarking or not embarking on a technologic intervention with medicine or machines. We are vigorously debating decisions about discontinuing those interventions when they are shown in individual cases not to be effective in "curing" the problem but only effective in preserving life. We must also consider how to allow individuals who do not require "heroic" medical intervention to die with dignity. Should they be allowed to commit suicide? Should we be able to help them die?

If you wish to support euthanasia, to what moral theory are you appealing? Do you argue that people have the right to control their own lives, and that euthanasia in these cases is like suicide—simply another instance of the right of self-determination? Would euthanasia enhance the well-being of either the individual or society? Would a euthanasia policy carry out the duty of society to respect individuals and their independence?

If you are opposed to euthanasia, what are the moral grounds of your opposition? Does it violate someone's right to life, even if the person renounces that right? Does it violate the respect we owe to a person? Does it violate our integrity to kill other people, no matter what the people killed think? Would a policy of euthanasia inevitably lead to abusive social practices?

Chapter 8

Rebecca

"This is the twenty-ninth meeting of the Care Review Committee. We are being asked by Dr. Goldstein for recommendations on his request to sterilize Rebecca Robinson, a 16-year-old retarded young lady. Dr. Goldstein, would you fill us in on this case?"

"Rebecca was referred to me by Dr. Kendig, who was formerly her pediatrician. She is a healthy young lady without any significant medical problems except migraine-like headaches. She is severely retarded, with an IQ measured at about 40. She has attended special classes in public schools and is very well socialized. She is pleasant, cooperative, takes care of herself in the simple ways, and is very attractive. She comes from a wonderful, caring family who have given her everything she needs. She goes on trips with them and fits in. She does need almost constant supervision because she lacks judgment and does not understand the consequences of her actions.

"The family came to me last summer after they had been to the beach with Rebecca. She had wandered off, and they found her on the edge of the park with a boy. Nothing serious happened, but they started thinking about what could have happened. They realized that Becky could get pregnant, and that there wasn't any way to prevent it except to keep her away from boys and under constant supervision. They came to me about birth control pills.

"I felt that they were contraindicated for Becky because of her migraine headaches, since there is a higher incidence of strokes in women with migraine who take oral contraceptives. Besides, Becky couldn't reliably take birth control pills on her own. We talked about IUDs and their problems and risks in adolescent girls. Her parents asked about tubal ligation. They raised the point, a good point, I thought, that they wanted Becky to be as normal as possible. They wanted her to have friends, including boyfriends. They wanted her to experience love, in whatever sense Becky could share it, but they didn't want her pregnant.

They are opposed to abortion on religious grounds, but for Becky they didn't see how she could be made to understand abortion even if they weren't opposed. They certainly didn't want her to go through pregnancy and delivery, which would be very traumatic to her. They also didn't want to raise another child or put one up for adoption. So the only alternative was to prevent pregnancy, and the best option was sterilization.

"I'm coming to the committee for your advice and consideration at the parents' request."

"What did you say was the cause of her retardation? Is it something that would affect a fetus?" asked Mrs. Adams.

"She has ideopathic retardation. We have found no cause and do not believe this is metabolic or genetic. She is a healthy young woman who could bear a normal infant. The reasons for requesting sterilization are psychological ones: the effects of the pregnancy on her and the problem of who would care for the child. Also to be considered are the restrictions that have to be imposed on her to prevent possible pregnancy. Clearly, Becky could not be responsible."

"Dr. Goldstein, could you tell us the risks of sterilization?"

"They are virtually negligible. It is an outpatient procedure, what we call band-aid surgery. A little local anesthesia, a laparoscopy, we find the tubes, put a clip on them, and that's all. She goes home the same day."

"I can't see any objection to this procedure," states Dr. Kendig. "I knew this family when I was Becky's pediatrician. They are extraordinary folks who have always done their best for her. That's why she's as good as she is today."

"I can see one objection," states Mr. Bacher, the hospital attorney. "It's illegal! She's 16 and can't give informed consent on the basis of her age, and no one can give informed consent for her. If this were a life-threatening condition or for her medical benefit, the parents could consent, but it's not. Parents and surgeons have been sued over sterilization of minors and lost! I'm not going to have this hospital sued. No way!"

"Couldn't they go to court and ask the judge for permission just as they do for blood transfusions for Jehovah's Witnesses?"

"They could," replies Bacher. "But no court would give permission to sterilize minors. Judges have been sued as well. You have to wait until she's 21, of legal age, and then get her permission."

"That's ridiculous!" shouts Kendig. "She won't be any more competent at 21 than she is now. Do you think her retardation will improve? At 21 the courts will have to declare her incompetent and give permission. Why can't they do it now? What's the family supposed to do for the next 5 years, keep her locked up? Or should Becky wear a chastity belt?"

"Well," says Bacher, "it's not clear that the judge would even give consent when she is 21. A judge was personally sued for allowing sterilization on a 21-yar-old girl and lost. I'm not sure anyone would be willing to take the chance, not without a specific statute on the books. There are too many 'advocates' who want retarded children to be normal—and that includes having babies. There have been too many abuses in the past where girls have been sterilized who shouldn't have been."

"You mean that the retarded have the right to be normalized and to have children, and they have the right, but not the capability to decide *not* to have children, and no one has the right to decide for them?" asks Goldstein.

"I guess that sums it up pretty well," mumbles Bacher. "The law only reflects society. If you want a different policy you're going to have to get the legislature to pass a law. I doubt they'd touch this issue with a ten-foot pole."

"Okay," says Dr. Thorne, the committee chairman. "This committee is not here to work out the legalities and practicalities of issues; we're here to assure that the right thing is done. Would one of you outline the ethical aspects of this situation? See if we could develop some guidelines for situations like this and some recommendations for Dr. Goldstein and Becky's parents."

* * *

Outline Becky's rights and how they are best protected. Does Rebecca have the right to love? Does she have the right to relationships with boys? Is this part of normalization? Does she have the right to sexual intercourse? Does she have the right *not* to get pregnant? How would she exercise that right, since she cannot use common forms of contraception?

Does sterilization violate her rights? Would it violate her right to bear children? Should the retarded have the right to bear children? Does the right to bear children carry with it responsibilities for those children? If the retarded child cannot assume those responsibilities, does she still have the right to have a child? Would you make the same arguments for an intellectually normal 14-year-old? How would you restrict her right?

Do Becky's parents, who have assumed the responsibilities for her care, upbringing, and supervision, have rights? Do they have the right to shelter her from pregnancy, labor, and delivery? Do they have the right to either mandate or refuse abortion if she were to become pregnant? What about adoption? Do they have the right not to raise another child? If the parents had assumed less responsibility for her development and placed her in an institution, would they have less right to supervise her activity? Or only less need to supervise it? If her parents do not have the right to exercise this control over Becky, who does?

Would subjecting Becky to the long-term risks of oral contraceptives or IUDs further her rights? Would sterilization lessen the risks?

Does refusing to sterilize Becky curtail more of her rights than sterilization?

Are rights dependent on IQ? Would her rights be different if her IQ were ten points higher? Twenty points? Thirty points? How valid are IQ tests?

Would a utilitarian approach make better decisions for Becky?

How would you weigh the benefits and costs of sterilization for Becky against the risks and benefits of: (1) constant supervision; (2) lifelong contraceptives; (3) pregnancy, labor, and delivery; (4) abortion; (5) keeping the infant at home, and (6) placing the infant for adoption?

How would you weigh the similar costs and benefits for Becky's parents? For society? At what level of intelligence would you find that your analysis would weigh against sterilization?

In a utilitarian fashion, how do you weigh the fact that Becky's sterilization would be against the law?

What would be the costs and benefits of breaking the law for Becky? For her parents? For society? For you? For your hospital? If the costs to you include a substantial risk of prosecution and even loss of your license, how would you, as a utilitarian, decide on what is best for Becky?

Are there other ethical approaches that would provide a basis for making better decisions for Becky?

Devise a process that would provide maximum protection for all parties concerned. How should Becky be involved? The parents? The physician? Society? Would an elaborate process add to or diminish Becky's rights?

Chapter 9

Christie

You are the chief resident in pediatrics at University Hospital. It is 9 P.M., and you are just signing out when the call comes. An obstetrician from Suburban Hospital is on the line. She has just attended the birth of a baby girl with spina bifida. The family practice residents are working with the baby now, but there is no crisis. The child did not need resuscitation in the delivery room. When can the child be transferred to University? You agree to take the child first thing in the morning and sign out for the night.

The emergency room calls at 9 A.M. to say that the ambulance from Suburban has arrived, and you tell them to send the baby up to the floor. You call the neurosurgical service, and the resident promises to come over. About ten minutes later the ambulance attendant wheels an isolette onto the floor. You sign the transfer papers and wheel the child into an examining room. The child is lying on her abdomen and appears perfectly normal. You lift her blanket and remove the sterile dressing from the cyst on her back.

The cyst is about the size of a tangerine and has some of the same color. It sits in the center of her lower back. Its surface is mottled red and yellow and flesh colored, but it seems to be intact. There is no apparent leak of spinal fluid and, therefore, no ready opening for infection. You measure the circumference of the child's head at 39 centimeters, a little above normal, so you know that there is some buildup of fluid in the head (i.e., hydrocephalus). The neurosurgical resident joins you, and together you begin to examine the child's legs to see what damage has been done to her motor functions. From the first, it does not look good. Both feet are clubbed; that is, they are turned in so that the soles face each other. This almost certainly means that the muscles that hold the feet in line have not developed because the nerves that control them are not functioning. It also means that the child will probably have her ankles in casts for her first six months, followed by an operation or two to

81

straighten each foot. You and the neurosurgical resident pinch the child's legs and chest. You pull her legs out and push them back. Finally, you stroke her legs and chest with an open safety pin. You are unable to get any motion in either of her legs, and she responds to the pin only from her abdomen up. This means that she is paralyzed from the waist down.

Spina bifida is a result of the failure of the neural tube, the tube that is to become the spinal cord, to close completely. Closure normally happens in the sixth to eighth week of pregnancy. On the basis of your examination, you now know that the spinal cord has been injured at the T10-12 level, the bottom level of the thoracic spine. All the nerves that leave the spinal column below that point, the nerves that branch off from the lumbar and sacral spine, are not functioning. This means that the child is paralyzed from the waist down and that she lacks sensation in both legs. It also means that the nerves that control her bladder and bowel functons are not working. She will need help in urinating and defecating. Her bladder is particularly important, since a buildup of urine in the bladder can back up into the kidneys and damage them.

Spina bifida is not an inherited disease, nor does it have a distinctive genetic pattern. Even though it occurs somewhat more frequently in certain ethnic groups and in some families, there are no exact ways of predicting its occurrence. It can be detected before birth through an analysis of aminotic fluid coupled with a careful ultrasound examination. Apart from the few couples who have had a previously affected child and whose future children are at special risk for the condition, it is hard to define a population at high enough risk for the condition to justify widespread screening programs.

The neurosurgical resident says, "What a damn shame. These kids have such a miserable life. I hope she doesn't linger on too long. That's always hard. You're surely not going to treat her."

You look away from him and say, "I don't know. There is nothing we can do to correct the paralysis, but there is a lot we can do to minimize its effects. With special braces she will be able to walk a little, at least until her teenage years. After that, of course, she'll be stuck in a wheelchair and she will have to work hard to keep from getting pressure sores."

The neurosurgical resident comes back, "But the physical handicaps are not the half of it. With even this mild hydrocephalus, she probably has a 10- to 20-percent chance of being retarded. We'll need to install a shunt to pass the extra fluid from her brain into her abdomen, and then she may need many operations to unclog the thing when it plugs, not to mention replacing it when she outgrows it. The whole business is just more than anyone should have to take. What quality of life is that? Shunt surgery takes its toll and increases the chance of her getting meningitis.

And then what would you have? A retarded child stuck lifelong in a wheelchair. No one would want to live that kind of life. Why not let nature take its course? Just leave her on the ward, give her standard care, and wait for that cyst to spring a leak. Her spinal fluid will then get infected. The infection will travel to her brain, and she will soon be dead of meningitis. It's the most humane thing to do."

"Well," you reply, now acutely conscious of the head nurse who has joined the group, "that way makes it really tough on the staff. They are not used to sitting around waiting for a baby to die, especially when there are things that could be done. Furthermore, the baby may not die, at least not any time soon. Of course, no one has really good numbers on it, but I bet that no more than 60 percent of these kids die if they get decent nursing care. Some of them don't develop meningitis, and others fight off the infection by themselves. And then you have a real disaster on your hands. You've let the hydrocephalus go, so you have a 2-year-old with an enormous head, certainly retarded, and destined for a long, slow death."

The neurosurgeon turned his head as he left the room, saying, "Well, are you going to treat the patients or are you going to treat the staff?"

But dealing with the nurse was no easier. "I'm glad to see you standing up for us," she said. "Fine," you reply, "but how would you answer the question? Are we really doing this kid a favor to treat her? Or are we just sentencing her to a long, dull life, or even a life full of nothing but one treatment or surgery after another? Sure there are some things we could do, but the fact that we can do them doesn't mean that we should. Granted that many of these handicapped kids do very well, some of them do very poorly, and we end up regretting ever starting on treatment."

"Well, I'm not sure how I feel about it," the nurse replies, "but you know that we could be reported under the 'Baby Doe' regulations for withholding medical treatment. And I don't want a bunch of people from downtown putting their noses in our business."

"I am not sure what I want to do either. Where's the father?"

"He's in the lounge. I'll get him, the social worker, and one of the other residents. We can all meet in the Parents' Lounge to decide. But you'll have to make the presentation to the father."

What are *you* going to say? You must decide how to present this material. You caught a glimpse of the father as the isolette was wheeled in. He has plainly been up all night. You see in the chart that he is a factory worker, so he probably does not know too much about biology, medicine, or handicapped children. You will need to start your explanations from the very beginning. How will you approach him? There are many possible approaches, and myriad gradients within each. We offer three for you to choose from.

Approach A: Your child has a very severe handicap. While there are some things we can do, we cannot solve her basic problems. It is unfair to sentence anyone to that kind of handicapped life. It would be a lot less cruel and there would be less suffering if she died soon. If we leave her alone, there is a good chance that is just what will happen.

Approach B: Although your child is very handicapped, and although we cannot correct the basic problems, there is a lot we can do to help her lead a happy, full life. Most handicapped people do, especially if they get first-rate care from the start. Let's give her a chance. Besides, there's no guarantee that not treating her will end in a quick and painless death.

Approach C: We are going to let you, the parents, decide. We will lay out the facts and the choices as best we can. But that's all we can do. Since she is your child, you and your wife will have to decide her fate. In this case, we can live with whatever you decide.

Carefully consider which approach you will take. Now that you have made your decision, but before it is irrevocable, consider the following points.

1. Whose decision is this?
- Is this the parents' decision? Will they be making an informed decision? How will the bias of your presentation influence their decision? Are they entitled to an additional presentation by someone with a different bias? Will the information overload of your presentation to this fatigued and overwhelmed father be improved by another presentation with a different bias?
- Can you live with whatever decision the parents make?
- Is this a physician (or medical staff) decision? Can you make the presentation so that the family will do whatever you think proper? Should you?
- Is this a social decision? Have the recent child abuse amendments mandated that all these children be treated? If so, why are you seeking consent from the parents? Or are you merely informing them?

2. Since your presentation will probably determine the parental decision, is there any philosophical theory that tells you what you should say?
   • Does the child have the right to treatment? If every infant has a right to treatment, does this mean they should all be treated? Does the child have the right to die?
   • Which decision will provide the greatest benefit for the child? Which decision will provide the greatest benefit for the parents? For society? How would you resolve potential conflicts among these benefits?

On the basis of further reflection, do you want to change the tenor of your presentation? Remember, you can never take back the impression your presentation makes on this father. The decision about how you present the material may be the most important decision you make in this case.

Now choose one of several approaches to the parents.

Approach A: You bias your presentation against treating the infant. Continue with the next section entitled "Approach A."

Approach B: You bias your presentation toward treating the infant. Turn to page 87.

Approach C: You believe that a physician should give as unbiased a presentation as possible. Therefore you present just the facts in as neutral a fashion as possible and leave the decision to the parents. Turn to page 89.

Approach A

"Mr. Boone, I'm Dr. Bradstreet, the chief resident in pediatrics, and I'm in charge of handling your daughter's case. What have you been told so far about her condition?"

"Well, last night at Suburban, all they said was that the baby has a very severe problem, but only the doctors at University could tell how bad it really was and what could be done."

"And how is your wife?"

"She's okay. Pretty weepy about the baby, but she'll be fine."

"Well, Mr. Boone, I'm afraid I have some bad news for you. Your baby has spina bifida, or open spine. This is a birth defect that happens very early, as the baby's spine is forming. Your baby is paralyzed from the waist down. There is nothing that we, or anyone else, can do to reverse that. We can use braces, if she is intelligent enough, and help her to hobble from place to place. But she will never really walk, and before adolescence she will be confined to a wheelchair for the rest of her life.

"In addition, your baby probably has water on the brain. We call it hydrocephalus. This occurs in most spina bifida babies, and it requires a shunt to prevent the buildup of fluid within the brain that can cause her head to swell to the size of a watermelon. The shunt is a small plastic tube that goes under the skin and drains the fluid into the stomach. Unfortunately, these tubes often get clogged or infected and need to be fixed. Yesterday I admitted a little boy for his sixth shunt operation in the past four months. Some of these children are retarded even if the shunt works, but blockage and certainly infection make the retardation even worse.

"If she is in a wheelchair and retarded, there is nothing useful she'll be able to do. If she is in a wheelchair and not retarded, it may be worse because she will understand how much of life she is missing, how different she is from other girls. Twenty percent of these children are retarded, and many have less severe intellectual problems.

"As if that isn't enough, spina bifida always causes paralysis of the bowel and bladder, so these children can't be toilet trained. They are in diapers for years, wet and smelly. It's really sad.

"We could start with a simple operation to close that cyst on her back, but that doesn't cure anything; it would just decrease her chances of getting an infection—meningitis. If we close her back, then we really should start on the shunt business, fix the feet, get braces, and just continue forever. If we were successful and lucky, we'd end up with a girl in a wheelchair looking out the window at her classmates jumping rope. She'd probably have few friends. What quality of life is that? I wouldn't want to live that way, and I wouldn't want that for my daughter. If we don't operate, these children often die quickly without pain or suffering. Usually they die of meningitis or hydrocephalus.

"She's your daughter and the decision is up to you and your wife, but I know what I would want if she were mine. I'd want to start over again and have a healthy child.

"Do you have any questions? I know that we haven't explained everything, but we've probably said all you can understand at one time. You'll need to talk this over with your wife. Unfortunately, we can't wait too long for a decision. If you decide to treat, the surgeons would like to get started tomorrow morning."

* * *

Estimate your powers of persuasion. Are you confident that these parents will follow your recommendation? If you are, or if you are unsure, turn to "Ethics Committee" (p. 91). If you believe that the parents will want treatment anyway, turn to "The Three-Month Report: C" (p. 101).

Approach B

"Hi, Mr. Boone, sit down. I'm Dr. Bradstreet, the chief resident in pediatrics, and I'm in charge of your daughter's care. What have you been told so far about her condition?"

"Well, last night at Suburban, all they said was that the baby had a very severe problem, but that only the doctors at University could tell how bad it was and what could be done."

"And how is your wife doing?"

"She's okay. Pretty weepy about the baby, but she'll be fine."

"I can understand why you're so upset. This whole business is new to you, of course, but we have a lot of experience in dealing with these problems. Your baby has spina bifida, or open spine. You may never have heard of this condition before, but it is actually one of the most common severe birth defects. It happens to about one in 1000 babies. Because the baby's spinal cord has not formed properly, the nerves that make the muscles move are not normal and the baby is paralyzed from the waist down. There isn't anything we can do to cure her paralysis, but there are lots of things we can do to help your baby. As these children grow up, they can use braces and crutches to stand and even to get from place to place. However, as your daughter becomes an adolescent, she will probably be too heavy for braces and will have to use a wheelchair. Children and adults can do very well in wheelchairs. Sometimes these children get pressure sores from sitting all the time; when they do, we treat them. Most of the children we see go to regular schools. They are able to learn normally and get along well with other children.

"In addition to paralysis, your child has started to develop water on the brain. We call this hydrocephalus. It is a common complication of spina bifida because the fluid that is produced in the brain is blocked from flowing through its normal channels down the spine. We treat this by installing a shunt, a small plastic tube, to pass the fluid from the brain to the stomach area. Although this may sound terrible, it is really a common procedure. The shunt lies under the skin and is completely invisible. We have to fix the shunts from time to time because children outgrow them or because they get blocked or infected, but serious problems are rare.

"There is another problem we should mention. Because the nerves in her spine have not developed, your child will not have normal control over bowel and bladder functions. This is not a problem during infancy, of course, because all children are wearing diapers. We will check carefully to see that her urine does not back up and damage her kidneys. When she gets older, we can train her to take care of herself. Our little boys and girls manage themselves quite well and are usually clean and dry when they are in school.

"Our decision right now is about an operation on her back. We should remove the sac and close the opening so that your baby will be easier to handle and, even more important, so that she won't get an infection. As it is now, the sac could leak and meningitis, an infection of the brain, could set in. Then your baby would be in deep trouble.

"Of course, we need your permission for the operation, and you'll need to explain all this to your wife. But to give your little girl the best chance for a good life, we should go ahead as soon as possible. I know it is just my bias, but it is what I would want if it were my child. We must do this operation as soon as possible to avoid infection."

* * *

Estimate your powers of persuasion. Are you certain the father will follow your recommendation? If so, turn to "The Three-Month Report: B" (p. 100). If you are at all unsure that the parents will decide to treat, turn to "Ethics Committee" (p. 91).

Approach C

"Mr. Boone, I am Dr. Bradstreet, the chief resident in pediatrics. I am here to help you and your wife make a decision. What have you been told about your child's condition?"

"Well, the doctors at Suburban said that the baby had a problem, but they didn't know how bad it was or what could be done. They said that you would have to help us."

"And how is your wife?"

"She's okay. Pretty weepy about the baby, but she'll be fine."

"I'll start, then, by laying out the facts of your child's condition. Then I'll ask you to talk it over on the phone with your wife and tell me what you decide.

"Your baby has a condition called spina bifida, or open spine. It is a problem that has its origin very early in the pregnancy. There are three major problems that it produces.

"The first is paralysis. Your child is paralyzed from the waist down, and that is irreversible. While your child is still young, she will be able to get around with braces and crutches; as she grows up, she will be confined more and more to a wheelchair. People respond to handicaps like this in very different ways, and there is no way to tell how your daughter will turn out in this regard. Some become superachievers, while others just seem to fall apart.

"In addition to the paralysis, your baby has water on the brain—hydrocephalus. The brain produces fluid that flows through narrow channels in the brain and down the spinal cord. When there is a blockage in the flow, fluid builds up and puts pressure on the brain. With surgery we can shunt the fluid around the blockage and into the stomach area. In about half of the children, the shunts themselves run into problems and we have to fix them. If we have good luck with the shunt, however, there is about an 80- to 90-percent chance that your child's intelligence will not be impaired by the spina bifida or its complications.

"The third major problem area is your child's bowel and bladder control. The paralysis affects not only the nerves in her legs but also those that control her bowel and bladder functions. These, too, will never be normal. We can, when she is 5 or 6, show her some ways to control herself so that she may go to a regular school and join in some of the things that other children do.

"The important decision for you and your wife is whether we should perform an operation to close the cyst on her back. This is not a very complicated operation, but it is major surgery and it is serious. If we get rid of the cyst and close her back, we will begin a series of operations to take care of her hydrocephalus and get her feet and legs ready for braces. Once we perform this first operation, her life expectancy is essentially normal.

"If, however, you decide against surgery, there is a very good chance that the cyst on her back will rupture and that her spinal fluid will become infected. The infection will travel to her brain and she may die, painlessly, of meningitis. There is a chance, between 25 and 50 percent, that either she will not develop an infection or that she will fight it off by herself. By about six weeks her back will heal spontaneously. At that time, however, hydrocephalus may have done some damage to her brain. Possibly, she will be much worse off for our having delayed treatment.

"While some people say that all of these children must be treated, there are others who disagree. I've had parents who have made both decisions. I can live with either one. I believe strongly that you and your wife are the ones who are closest to the baby, and the ones who will have to care for her.

"The decision is yours. Although we haven't been able to explain everything, we've probably told you all you could absorb in so short a time. We really can't wait too long to make a decision. We should know by first thing tomorrow if you want us to operate."

* * *

What decision do you think the parents will make? Were you neutral because you thought that was the most appropriate position to take or because you didn't feel strongly?

That night the father calls you and is very confused. He asks for further advice. You refer them to the Ethics Committee. Turn to the following section.

Ethics Committee

If there is any thought of not treating a newborn in Christie's condition, federal regulations suggest, and the policies of many hospitals demand, that the matter be brought before a hospital ethics committee. The following is an account of how such a meeting might proceed.

"Thank you very much for coming, Doctor," begins John Thorne, M.D., assistant chief of the medical staff and chairman of the Infant Care Review Committee. "I am sure you have a basic idea of what we are about, but let me remind you of a few items. Our committee was created by the hospital in response to the Child Abuse Amendment of 1984 and the 1985 regulations implementing it. The hospital has charged us with helping physicians and parents to make decisions about appropriate care for seriously afflicted newborns. We are strictly an advisory group; we're not going to make this tough decision for you. Our job is to talk this case through, making sure you see all the sides and all the angles. Also, to put the matter bluntly, we try to keep the Child Protective Service Agency and its pushy social workers out of the hospital. We don't want anyone leveling charges of medical neglect or telling us how to practice medicine.

"Let me introduce the committee members from outside the hospital. At the far end of the table is Professor Scott Armstrong of the University's philosophy department. He is a consulting ethicist with us. Opposite him is Paul McBundy, the hospital's chief counsel. On my right is Mrs. Lucille Adams, chairman of the Right to Life Society. On my left is George Lear of the Council for the Disabled.

"Let me begin by reviewing the section of the current federal regulations that define medical neglect."

The term "withholding of medically indicated treatment" means the failure to respond to the infant's life-threatening conditions by providing treatment (including appropriate nutrition, hydration, and medication) which, in the treating physician's reasonable medical judgment, will be most likely to be effective in ameliorating or correcting all such conditions, except that the term does not include the failure to provide treatment (other than appropriate nutrition, hydration, or medication) to an infant when, in the treating physician's reasonable medical judgment, any of the following circumstances apply:

    i. The infant is chronically and irreversibly comatose;

    ii. The provision of such treatment would only prolong the dying, not be effective in ameliorating or correcting all of the infant's life-threatening conditions, or otherwise be futile in terms of the survival of the infant; or

    iii. The provisions of such treatment would be virtually futile in terms of the survival of the infant and the treatment itself under such circumstances would be inhumane.

Federal Register 50 (No. 72), April 15, 1985

"I shudder every time you read their bureaucratic gobbledygook. Before going further, let's get clear on the facts of this case," interrupted Mr. McBundy. "Dr. Thorne, would you please review the facts for the medical laity?"

At the conclusion of his review of the medical situation as presented on pages 81 and 82, Dr. Thorne added, "There's also the psychosocial picture. According to the unit social worker, the parents feel that Christie might be better off without all the surgery and they aren't sure they want her treated.

"Does anyone on the committee have any questions? Mr. McBundy."

"As an attorney I hate to admit this, but I don't see any issue here. What basis is there for not treating the child? She isn't dying; she isn't comatose; treatment wouldn't be futile or inhumane. The hospital and you doctors certainly don't want a bunch of folks from Protective Services, followed closely by the press, snooping around here and telling you what to do. The regulations talk about 'reasonable medical judgment.' Their guidelines for withholding treatment are clear enough, and this case doesn't fit within them."

"Well, Paul, as with all legal documents, it depends on how you read them," put in Dr. Goldsmith, a senior pediatrician on the staff. "I've examined the baby; in my reasonable medical judgment I don't think that leaving her alone would be medical neglect. If she gets meningitis, she's likely to die soon. Meningitis is a natural part of this condition. She is also dying of hydrocephalus. Dr. Lorber in England has published a number of impressive studies that show that these children, if untreated, die quickly. What's more, there is nothing medicine can do to correct the paralysis of the legs, bowel, and bladder or to treat any retardation. In that sense, therefore, treatment is futile. Also, since she'll be confined to a wheelchair, isolated from other kids and forced to spend long months in the hospital for orthopedic surgery and neurosurgery, treatment could well be inhumane. I think that catches all the buzzwords. You see, it isn't so clear.

"I agree with you that the key words are 'reasonable medical judgment.' But we've got two opinions here, one from a neurosurgeon and one from a pediatric consultant. Both physicians know about this case and about spina bifida. They agree about everything, even the statistics about outcome. They differ only about whether one should risk a bad outcome and the quality of a child's life with such a result. One recommends the surgery even though she recognizes the chance for a bad outcome. The other recommends against surgery although he, too, is ambivalent.

"Since reasonable medical judgments differ, no one could argue that there is a medically indicated treatment that is being withheld."

"Well," interrupted Mrs. Adams, "you doctors might be able to slip around with medical terminology and all your weasel words about 'reasonable judgment,' but there is something obvious here that is just staring you in the face. That little baby has rights. Even in the abominable Supreme Court decision granting a legal right to abortion, the Court declared that viable fetuses had a right to life. And that's what we're talking about here. A baby's life is at stake under all those mushy medical words. This is a life or death decision, not a nose job.

"Why don't you just face up to what you're thinking about? You want that baby dead because handicapped kids are a pain. You're just trying to let her die because she's not the kind of child you want. And none of you has the guts to say that she should be killed. 'Let nature take its course'—what nonsense when the whole point of this hospital and modern medicine is to change the natural course of a disease. You're just trying to cover up your murderous intentions.

"But there's a matter of rights here. Our society did not invest all it has in modern medicine just to save the cute and beautiful. All these children have rights, God-given rights in my view, but you can call them civil rights if you like. And they aren't just the rights of football players and pom-pom girls. Life is life—in braces, in a wheelchair, in bed, whatever. In our system, that right to life means the right to medical treatment. Depriving Christie of treatment, sentencing her to death, is a denial of her legally guaranteed rights. These rights are moral and legal absolutes, and they must not be abridged."

"It's not that easy, Lucille," said Mr. Lear quietly. "You haven't had to raise a handicapped child. I have. That's why I'm on this committee. My daughter is 15 now. At birth she was much like Christie. She is paralyzed from the waist down. We've had to give up on braces; she's been in a wheelchair for the last three years. Thank God her shunt hasn't been a lot of trouble. She's at the top of her class at Central High. But it hasn't been easy for us, or for Mary. She's our only child. We didn't think we could afford more, financially or emotionally. My wife gave up her career so Mary would get everything she needed.

"Also, all this medical care doesn't come cheap. And a lot of the wheelchairs, equipment, and therapy are not well covered, even by the best insurance policies. I'm not complaining; for us it's been worth it.

"Mary still has her problems. When the girls at school start talking about boys, Mary is left out. She tries to stay above it all, but I know she hurts a lot inside. She has only a few real friends. Her best friend is a girl with cerebral palsy. Mary spends a lot of time with us. We're a very close family, maybe even too close. I don't know if it's the wheelchair, the fact that she sometimes soils herself and smells, or just that she's different, but people are always staring at her when we go out. Is Mary happy? I don't know. She's brave and tries hard, but it's not the same as being a normal kid.

"And Mary is one of the lucky ones. At the meetings of the parent's group, I see children who aren't as bright, who don't have schoolwork to brag about, or whose families have split up under the pressure of caring for them. Some of the children are in foster homes, and many lack some kind of financial or emotional support.

"I don't know about the medical ambiguity, Lucille, but I can see the human ambiguity. Just because Christie has the right to treatment, and I think everyone recognizes that, doesn't mean that her parents should exercise that right for her. Just because you have the right of free speech doesn't mean that you should say something. We have to make a suggestion to these people whether or not they should play their trump card and have Christie treated. After all, adults have the right to refuse treatment they don't want. Christie, or somebody acting for her, should have the same right.

"Since you brought up the subject of rights, Lucille, I find it hard to fathom why some of your friends in the right to life groups, people so interested in the right to treatment, don't support the social programs that make that right a real option.

"Even if they had full support, however, I'm not sure it would be good enough for these kids. It isn't such an easy decision. Come to the parent's group sometime."

Putting down his pipe, Professor Armstrong began in his most patient tone of voice. "That's the whole problem with setting up the issue as a matter of rights. Everyone in our society likes to talk about rights, but such talk quickly degenerates into sloganeering. If we can't decide what rights people have, which rights have priority, and who decides which rights to use, all the talk about rights won't settle the moral issues. Furthermore, talking about rights immediately introduces moral absolutes that are philosophically very suspect.

"We need to think about the quality of Christie's life and the life of her family and the whole society. Thinking hard about the quality of the lives involved seems to me to be the only way to reach a good decision in the case.

"Let's look at the positive side first. Treatment brings a great increase in the chances of Christie's survival. Everyone will admit that is a benefit. She will bring some happiness and satisfaction to her parents—also a benefit. She could be of some service to society as a whole, but how much is impossible to estimate without better knowledge of her intelligence. Let's be conservative and put her down for only a small benefit to society. From everything we've heard so far, it is hard to think she will have a high quality of life. The quality may be good, perhaps adequate, but probably not high.

"The negatives are on the other side of the balance sheet. The costs to Christie are in a life of frustration, confinement, and discomfort. The cost to her parents are in their emotional well-being as parents of a handicapped child and the large monetary costs of Christie's care. Finally, the costs to society are enormous. Christie will be a constant drain on society's resources, yet the chance of her making a substantial contribution are very slight. She may lower the life quality of many other people.

"As I read the scales, therefore, the burdens of Christie's medical care are disproportionate to the benefits. The benefits are too meager to justify the enormous commitment, both on society's part and Christie's own part. I know I'll be accused of being too tough for thinking this way. In fact, although it is hardheaded, it is softhearted. It is really trying to add to the quality of the social and emotional lives of all concerned."

"Just a moment, now, Scott. I'm not convinced your method is even as hardheaded as you pretend," began Mr. McBundy. "As I remember my philosophy classes, the quality of life calculus you are proposing was criticized for being wishywashy and arbitrary. After all, Christie could be a great singer or a brilliant computer programmer. Then the benefits to herself, her family and, most of all, to society could be enormous. Toss that on the scale and watch the balance shift. What you put on the scales is very arbitrary, and you can always fiddle with the weights to get the answer you want. As I recall, there were a lot of philosophers who argued that proportional moral reasoning could be used to justify even such obvious atrocities as slavery.

"I always found myself more attracted to the Kantian theory, which is based on the respect that every person owes to every other. Just as we all want to be respected and treated as fully human beings, so we should treat others in the same way. Christie is no less of a person because of her age, sex, or physical handicap. If Christie were not handicapped, we wouldn't be having this meeting. Our duty to her would be clear, and we would be busy about her medical care. Well, our duty is clear; respect for Christie demands that we treat her. Anything else is dereliction of our duty and rank discrimination. This is the legal duty that I mentioned earlier, and also our moral duty."

"No one here is arguing for discrimination in that sense," said Dr. Goldsmith, shifting uneasily. "But good medical practice demands that we discriminate in a technical way. Christie *is* different from other kids; she has a substantial handicap. As I see it, common sense dictates that we should try to do what is best for her. But what is best seems very ambiguous. None of the formulas that have been proposed—calculating the benefits, recognizing rights, or doing our duty—are wholly persuasive. And the medical experts on the case are divided as well. In light of so much diversity, I don't see how the committee can make a definitive recommendation.

"I am content that we have shared our views with Christie's physicians, and they can pass them on to the parents. I hope the people most involved can sit down and work out a decision that is best for all concerned."

"I think you're right, Saul," added Dr. Thorne. "Now I know how Harry Truman felt when he prayed for a one-handed economist. On the one hand, people say this, then on the other hand, that. When you see all the hands, you are more confused than when you started.

"It wouldn't make any sense to vote on this case. We're all coming at it from different angles. However, our meeting provided a good sounding board for various points of view. I think there is no choice but to refer the decision back to those most directly concerned—Christie's parents and the doctors who are working with them."

*　*　*

Does ethical discussion inevitably end in an impasse in which each person presents a different point of view, but no resolution is achieved? Does the fact that no resolution is achieved mean that none is possible? Is there a right answer in medical-ethical situations such as this? Are there clearly wrong answers? Perhaps agreement should be sought about which answers are wrong.

As you work through the cases in this book, you should expect to develop more understanding of the ethical theories sketched by the characters in the Ethics Committee meetings. Even at this point, is there one theory with which you feel more comfortable? (Remember, that does not mean you feel comfortable with or in complete agreement with the character advocating the theory.) What seems to be the strength of the theory? What are its weaknesses? There is a more extensive discussion of ethical theory in Chapters 14 and 15.

Decide what you think should be done, and also how you think the parents will react. There are many possible combinations of parental wishes and physician response to their desires. Let us assume only three.

1. The parents decline treatment and you go along with their decision.
2. You and the parents decide to treat Christie.
3. The parents decide to treat Christie and, despite your misgivings, you acquiesce.

Write a note to the Ethics Committee thanking them for their time and explaining the disposition of Christie's case. As far as possible, justify your stance explicitly in terms of an ethical theory. How do you deal with Christie's rights, with what is best for her, with the cost of her treatment, and with the duties of physicians and her parents?

After preparing this note, turn to the pages indicated to see how the case develops. If you took possibility 1, turn to "The Three-Month Report: A" (below). If you took possibility 2, turn to "The Three-Month Report: B" (p. 100). If you took possibility 3, turn to "The Three-Month Report: C" (p. 101).

The Three-Month Report: A

After much thought and consultation, the parents decide not to have surgery performed to close Christie's back and take her home.

Christie is now three months old, and the family has finally agreed to bring her in to see you. She is doing very well. Her back healed over, minimizing the chance of her getting meningitis. The cyst on her back is now simply an inconvenience to her parents in taking care of her. Christie's legs are still spindly and paralyzed, and nothing has been done to correct her clubbed feet.

Christie went home with her parents after two weeks in the hospital. She remained in the hospital only until her mother could get home and adjust. After about two weeks at home, Christie developed a slight fever and seemed dull and sluggish. In a phone conversation with the parents, you suggest that this was possibly meningitis. Considering the decision that was made, you did not want to examine the baby and document the infection. Christie recovered without medical intervention. At three months she is lively and alert. She gurgles and responds with a social smile. There is no evidence at this point that her development is delayed, although it is much too early to say much about her future intelligence.

Christie does, however, have a problem, and another decision point has been reached. The hydrocephalus noted at birth has progressed, and Christie's head is becoming noticeably large. The pressure on her brain will soon cause irreparable damage, if it hasn't already. If Christie is to die, it will now probably be from hydrocephalus, and this is a far less peaceful way to go than meningitis in infancy. In the months or years before she dies, her head will become so large and so heavy that carrying her around will be difficult. She will be completely unable to move herself. Residential institutions will not care for her in this condition. They will insist that a shunt be installed, but by that stage she will be retarded and probably blind.

No matter the original decision and whether you agreed with it, you are convinced that Christie has "passed the test of life." She is unlikely now to get meningitis, and you believe that slow death from hydrocephalus is medically and morally unacceptable. She is a smiling, bright, little baby. You believe that the time has come to treat her vigorously before her hydrocephalus worsens. The parents, however, are not at all convinced. Mr. Boone, with the clear agreement of his wife, does the talking.

"You know, Dr. Bradstreet," he begins, "Christie's birth has been real upsetting to us. We felt when she was first born that we must have done something wrong. Well, Sarah, my wife, has this friend who has tried to get us into this group for a long time. Since Christie was born, a lot of the things this lady has been saying began to make sense, and now we know that it was the kind of stuff we were eating that was the cause of Christie's problems.

"Thinking about that has not made us feel very good, but our friend says that right eating can cure the very problems that bad eating made. What Christie needs is nerve food, so we've added special seaweed and raw fish to her diet. Of course, that's all that Sarah is eating so the baby is getting it in her nursing, also. We are now pretty sure that all your operations and your pills aren't going to help Christie. Even from what you've said, they're not going to heal the nerves in her back, and they're not going to give her normal intelligence either, are they?"

"No," you have to say. "Our treatment will not heal the nerves in her spine. There is no way to guarantee Christie's intelligence. It looks like she has normal intelligence now, but if we don't take the pressure off her brain, we can guarantee that she will end up very retarded. I am not complaining about Christie's diet, and I'm not saying it won't work, but I am saying that we've got to use standard medical practice to get the extra fluid off her brain and into her stomach where it can be absorbed and passed off."

"Is this just one operation you're talking about?" Christie's dad continued. "And how much medicine and poison are involved?"

"If we're lucky, one operation will do it. But I wouldn't be honest if I didn't tell you that better than half the children require more than one operation, and some require several. The shunt tubing may become blocked or infected, and we would have to go in and fix it."

"And if you do all this, will Christie be normal?"

"There is no way to guarantee that Christie will have a normal intelligence. But, I have to repeat, if we don't operate, we can guarantee that she will be seriously retarded."

"Well, then, doctor, we don't see how we can go along with that operation. We've thought about this a long time and, thanks to our friend, we've looked up a lot of information on the subject. You can't guarantee that your methods will work, and we thank you for being up front about that. We think Christie has a better chance with right eating. We've seen a difference since we've started this. She wasn't even smiling when we began. And now a stay in the hospital and all the poisons you'll give her, not to speak about the food, will just set her back.

"Thank you, doctor, but no. We don't think you can give what Christie needs. We'll call you if we change our minds."

Despite further efforts to convince Christie's parents to allow treatment, they continue to refuse. You must decide whether to accuse them of medical neglect and to ask the state's Department of Child Protective Services to grant the hospital temporary custody of Christie. The hospital's attorneys have assured you that there will be no trouble getting a court order in this case. You are not sure, however, how the parents will respond. They clearly love Christie very much, but the group to which they now belong condemns the use of antibiotics and other drugs as polluting. Will they still be so caring of their daughter after she has become tainted by your treatment?

* * *

Before you decide whether or not to go to court, there are some things you should consider.

99

1. Is this really medical neglect? Or is it just your bias that rejects nonstandard medical practice? Do the family's obvious concern, love, and good intentions affect your decision?
2. Who is the best advocate for the child? You, the caring parents, or a guardian appointed by the court?

After thinking about these questions, choose one of the following options. If you decide to get a court to order treatment, turn to "The Three-Year Report: W" (p. 101). If you decide not to force her parents to have her treated, turn to "The Three-Year Report: X" (p. 103).

The Three-Month Report: B

The parents decide to have Christie's back closed. She is now three months old and spent the first eight weeks of her life in the hospital. In this time she had a number of operations.

After her back was surgically repaired on the second day of life, focus shifted to her hydrocephalus. Her head seemed to be growing at close to a normal rate, so an operation did not seem necessary. However, at three weeks of age the head began to grow quickly, and the surgeons were asked to install a shunt. They did this without complication. Now, however, at the second checkup since her discharge, it is plain that the shunt is not working well. Christie is listless, and examining the shunt shows that it is not working properly. She will have to come into the hospital to see whether the shunt can be fixed or to have a new shunt installed.

Her bladder and kidneys also are not doing well. Studies of kidney function reveal that there is a backup of urine, and she may be sustaining kidney damage. Her persistent low fever is probably caused by a urinary tract infection. The usual antibiotics have not done the job, so cultures will have to be prepared, the bug identified, and the proper medication chosen. Further tests will determine whether surgery is needed to correct what could be a long-term kidney problem.

At least you hope that the urinary tract is the source of the infection. If, however, the fever is due to an infection associated with the shunt, the problems could be complicated and severe. They could take weeks of hospitalization to straighten out and could end by causing retardation or even death.

Now is not the time to turn back in Christie's care. The point here is to recognize that, even though you have given her the most dedicated medical care, there is no assurance that Christie will do well.

The decisions to be made at this point are primarily medical. There is no good way to predict how they will come out. The decision you and Christie's parents made at the beginning has had an unexpected but not unusual outcome. To emphasize the unpredictable character of decisions in such cases, flip a coin to see what Christie will be like at 3 years of age. If the coin comes up heads, turn to "The Three-Year Report: Y" on page 104. If the coin comes up tails, turn to "The Three-Year Report: Z" on page 105.

The Three-Month Report: C

After much thought and consultation, the parents decide to have Christie's back closed and her hydrocephalus shunted.

At three months Christie is doing extremely well. She is a bright, alert, and happy baby. She seems to be developing normally, except for the paralysis in her legs. Her parents are delighted with her, and all their family and friends are supportive. Christie left the hospital after six weeks. Her hydrocephalus is under control after her shunt at two weeks of age. Fortunately, there have been no problems so far. Checking her bladder and kidneys reveals no damage, and Christie's parents and even her grandparents have learned to catheterize her. The orthopedic surgeons are getting ready to work on Christie's feet, but she seems little bothered by the casts she has been wearing.

At this point, Christie is a medical success. To find more about her outcome, flip a coin. If the coin comes up heads, turn to "The Three-Year Report: Z" on page 105. If the coin comes up tails, turn to "The Three-Year Report: Y" on page 104.

The Three-Year Report: W

Although there is no "final outcome" in a case of this sort, an assessment at 3 years of age provides a good indicator of her future prospects.

As you anticipated 2½ years ago, the court ordered Christie treated, and the treatment was medically successful. Christie is a reasonably bright and alert little girl. She is on schedule, or a little ahead, in her developmental milestones. There are no signs of kidney damage. She is adjusting well to her braces. She is able to stand and is beginning to take a few steps. But Christie, her foster mother says, is a very unhappy little girl.

Christie's parents were deeply hurt by the hearing in court. The media picked up the story, and there was wide public discussion of the "crazy" parents. Christie's father seemed particularly vulnerable to the pressure and, after a few months, he disappeared, abandoning Christie and her mother. Meanwhile, the nutrition and diet group with which they had affiliated began to break apart. When Christie was about 1 year old, her mother had a spell of deep depression during which she threatened to harm Christie. The social worker noticed suspicious red marks on Christie's arms and legs and had the child committed to protective custody. Christie's mother has taken her back for brief periods, but she is plainly not stable enough to care for her. Christie has been in three different homes, and the present one seems to be doing a good job. Christie's foster mother is very concerned about her emotional condition, but Christie's mother is not strong enough to take her back, nor is she willing to put her up for adoption. Although Christie is a medical success, you fear she is rapidly becoming a social disaster. Would Christie now be better off if you had urged treatment from the very beginning and obtained a court order, if necessary, to do it? Christie might have been at least as well off medically, and presenting the family with little or no option might well have pulled this fragile family together. Perhaps giving her parents so much choice was unfair to Christie and not a particular service to her parents. Or was the court-ordered treatment a mistake? Would Christie be better off untreated?

To get a picture of Christie untreated, turn to the next section.

What went wrong? As you think back about this case, would you have made different decisions? Such reflection is often conducted in real life. At least here, if you wish, you can go back to the beginning and try again.

If not, turn to the "Conclusion" at the end of this chapter.

The Three-Year Report: X

Although there is no "final outcome" in a case of this sort, an assessment at 3 years of age provides a good indication of her future prospects. Two and a half years ago you decided not to get a court to order treatment, and Christie is now a medical and social services disaster.

The burden of taking care of Christie turned out to be overwhelming for her parents. Her father seemed particularly vulnerable to the pressure and, after a few months, he disappeared, abandoning Christie and her mother. Meanwhile, the nutrition and diet group became discouraged with Christie's lack of progress and began to accuse her mother of cheating on the recommended foods. Christie's mother became depressed and separated from the group. Christie's constantly enlarging head was noticed by the neighbors, and a child abuse complaint was filed to allow the intervention of the state's Department of Social Services. The social worker placed Christie in protective custody, and, when she was 1 year old, a judge ordered medical treatment for her. A shunt was placed and was then replaced several times. Her cerebral spinal fluid persistently clogs the shunt. Christie's mother has taken her back for brief periods, but she is plainly not stable enough to care for her. Christie has been in three different foster homes, and the present one seems to be doing a good job. How long they will be able to continue to care for this severely impaired child remains to be seen.

In Christie's case medical intervention was too late to correct her problems. Her hydrocephalus was too advanced for a shunt to be effective. Christie is profoundly retarded. She has lost her vision and, although she startles at a noise, she does not really hear sounds. Her head is the size of a small watermelon. For the immediate future, the greatest danger to Christie's life comes from the bedsores she develops on her head because she is not able to move.

Her kidneys have been damaged by the backup of urine, but her present foster home is careful about catheterizing her so the damage is not great. Christie can live for a long time in this condition, but it does not seem to be much of a life.

Are you pleased with the outcome of your decisions?

Would Christie now be better off if you had urged treatment from the very beginning and filed a child neglect complaint, if necessary, to do it?

Christie would almost certainly be better off medically. Presenting the family with little or no option might well have pulled this fragile family together. Perhaps giving them so much choice was both unfair to Christie and no particular service to her parents.

In real life physicians often reflect on an outcome that turns out badly. Would you make the same decision again? If you think you should have asked for a court order at three months, turn back to "The Three-Year Report: W" on page 101. Unlike real life, here you can go back and start again. After following several paths, turn to the "Conclusion" at the end of this chapter.

The Three-Year Report: Y

Although there is no "final outcome" in a case of this sort, an assessment at 3 years of age provides a good indication of her future prospects. Christie is a bright and alert little girl. She is a little above average in making her developmental milestones. She is very verbal and a little precocious. There are no signs of kidney damage and her bowel movements are well controlled by diet. She is adjusting well to her braces. She is able to stand and is beginning to take a few steps. She is clearly a medical success.

Christie's family has responded wonderfully to the challenge of her care. Their family life is, if anything, stronger because of her. They have a second child now. Their newborn son does not have spina bifida and is a distraction from the perhaps excessive attention they were paying to Christie. While there are no guarantees, the medical and social prognosis for Christie is excellent.

Are you pleased with the outcome of your decision? You shouldn't be. Remember, the outcome was determined by the flip of a coin. If you are pleased, go to the next section to see the other possible outcome. In any event, go back through the case and examine several other options. If you have not done so, be sure to read the discussion of the Ethics Committee on page 91. Finally, turn to "Conclusion" at the end of the chapter.

The Three-Year Report: Z

Although there is no "final outcome" in a case of this sort, an assessment at 3 years of age provides a good indication of her future prospects. Christie has not done well medically or socially.

While Christie is not a medical success, neither is she a disaster. She is behind in her developmental milestones and, although it is still too early to be sure, she is probably mildly retarded (IQ = 75). Her kidneys have sustained some damage from the backup of urine, but they are still functioning. She has had innumerable bladder infections, some even re-quiring hospitalization. Her feet have been surgically straightened, and she now wears full leg braces. She is able to stand with the braces, but she has not been able to maneuver them so as to walk.

The greatest obstacles to her development at this point come from her social situation. Although home life went quite well at the start, Christie's father found the pressure of caring for her more and more of a burden. When she was about 1 year old, he disappeared, abandoning Christie and her mother. At that time her mother became very depressed and, among other things, threatened to abuse Christie. Christie was placed in a foster home for a while and has been returned to foster care several times since. Her medical care has been irregular over the past 2 years. Care of Christie is a great burden for her mother and both of them seem discouraged and demoralized. It is hard to tell what to make of their future.

What went wrong? As you think back about this case, would you have made different decisions? Such reflection is often conducted in real life. At least here, if you wish, you can go back to the beginning and try again. After following several paths, including a visit with the Ethics Committee on page 91, turn to the "Conclusion" on the next page.

Conclusion

If your decision turned out well, should you now be congratulating your-self? How much of the outcome depended on your decision? If your decision turned out badly, should you resolve to make a different decision in future spina bifida cases? Bad results might equally be due to bad luck.

Think about the problems that the unpredictability of result raises for the morality of decisions. Is unpredictability of outcome just a technical problem that could be overcome by better decision theory, or is it a problem for any moral theory that tries to evaluate actions on the basis of their consequences? If you find that outcome is not decisive in determining the morality of actions, you might think further about moral theories based on duties, or rights, or virtues. What moral theory most adequately deals with uncertainty?

Review your decision-making process at each step in this case and consider whether your decisions were morally sound. If you based your decisions on a different theory, would you have made better decisions? Would they have come out differently? Try going through the case basing your decision on utilitarian models, on rights, or on obligations. Does one feel better than another? Do they lead to different outcomes?

Comment

The presentation of Christie does not do justice to the many alternative decisions possible in a case of spina bifida. If the parents decided not to treat, you could have obtained a court order for treatment and had Christie adopted by a caring family. If, on the other hand, you agreed with their decision, the child might have died and the family might then have had other, normal children. If you and the parents had been enthusiastic about treatment, the infant might have done well, or badly, or somewhere in between. However, at the time of the initial decision, neither you, the family, the committee, nor the courts can accurately predict the outcome for any of the involved parties.

Chapter 10

The Smyth Saga

"Robert? are you asleep yet, dear? The dance tonight for all those poor children. . . . I really think I'd like to be more involved with a charity like that. Maybe with my advertising background I could be of some help."

"Hum?"

"I don't know what I'd do if I had to cope with a handicapped child. Maybe we shouldn't have children. Maybe we're too old, too settled in our professional lives. Do you think so? But then I think of my niece, Amy—she's so precious, so cute. It would be fun. I'd even cut back my work at the agency for one like that. I've been thinking about going to that Pregnancy Counseling Center and seeing what they have to say. Would you come with me?"

"Darling, we're not getting married until September. Do we have to make a decision tonight?"

"Of course not. Good night, sweet."

"You're 32, Virginia, and in good health. Is that correct? Any problems in your family? No? Your mother is now 57 and in good health. Your father is 60 and well. One sister, 27, and she has just one daughter. I see you have no children by your first marriage? Okay. Well, Virginia, was there a specific problem you had in mind? Your family history looks pretty clean. You are getting a bit older, but not to the age where Down's syndrome becomes a significant risk. If you are really concerned, we could do an amniocentesis early in your pregnancy—when and if you get pregnant—but we can only look for specific abnormalities such as Down's syndrome, so even amniocentesis doesn't guarantee a healthy baby. However, your risks are very small, no greater than anyone else's. Are there any special problems on your fiancé's side of the family? Why don't you check? If there aren't, I don't think you have much to worry about. Why don't you make another appointment if you have special concerns or when you're pregnant, but do it early in the pregnancy."

"This is one of my favorite restaurants, Robert. I think I'll have the veal again. Thank goodness for expense accounts. I went to the Pregnancy Counseling Center today and the counselor told me not to worry, that 32 wasn't too old and that there was nothing in my family to worry about. She said to ask about your side. Do you have anything hidden I don't know about, dear?"

"Only my Uncle Charles, with two heads. Or is it two personalities? Good Puritan stock. Dad has only the one brother, and his kids are fine, and my two children you know. I guess that's it. I'll ask my father if there's anything if you want me to. Now that I think about it, I think Dad had a sister who died; I'll ask him."

"Look, Virginia, lay off. It seems to be all you've got on your mind these past two weeks. I'll tell you one more time. All Dad knew was that his sister got rheumatic fever or chorea or something in her 30s; it got worse and drove her crazy. She ended up in a mental institution. She was much older than he was, so he doesn't remember the details. That's it. Now you've got Uncle Charles' wife all stirred up about his Parkinsonism. What's this about Huntington's disease, anyway? What is it, and what's it go to do with us?"

"Robert, don't get so upset. This is important, dear. Just take a look at this pamphlet about Huntington's disease that I picked up today at the Center. Could this be what your aunt had? I've underlined the important parts. It's very frightening—maybe for you, and even for our children."

Huntington's Disease—The Terrible Killer

Huntington's disease is a progressive degenerative disease characterized by changes in personality, and the gradual onset of a disorder of movement leading to progressive intellectual deterioration and death. While occasionally taking a different and more severe form in childhood, it usually begins in the third, fourth or fifth decades of life with subtle alterations in movements—sometimes thought to be tics. These progress over several years. The movements may precede the intellectual deterioration or follow subtle intellectual and emotional changes. The movements and intellectual problems gradually become so severe that the individuals are unable to care for themselves. These individuals often spend their last years in a nursing home or institution. Huntington's disease is an autosomal dominant trait. Each child of an affected parent has a 50 percent chance of having the disease, even if the disease is not visible in the parent. Every person who carries the gene will pass it on to 50 percent of their children. Thus, many families have elected not to have children.

There is no known therapy. That is why we need your help and your funds for research to help stamp out this terrible disorder.

The Huntington's Disease Committee

"That's grim," states Robert. "Terrific bedtime reading, but what's it got to do with us?"

"Well, yesterday I was talking with your Aunt Libby. Charles' doctor had been asking them about diseases in the family. It seems that Charles' Parkinsonism isn't behaving the way it's supposed to and the name Huntington's disease came up. They were asking how his father died, his mother, and then this sister. Her death seemed to intrigue them. Charles said your father has all that information since he was the lawyer for the estate. You know, I don't believe Charles' mind is as sharp as it used to be."

"Yes, Dr. Gunderson," Mr. Smyth replies, "I know quite a bit about Huntington's disease. That is how my sister died. She was about 50 when she passed away. An autopsy was done; I have the report. . . . No, I haven't told anyone in the family. There didn't seem to be much point, and I don't think that you should tell the others either. I want to emphasize that this is a confidential conversation between you and me. Let me explain.

"When Mary died, Charles already had two young children and wasn't planning to have more. Robert was 10, and my wife and I had already decided not to have more children. Charles was always a hypochondriac—rushing off to doctors with each little ache or pain—so there didn't seem to be much reason to lay the burden of Mary's diagnosis on him and add to his concerns. Besides, Charles had a 50-percent chance of not having it. My father had died in an automobile accident in his early 50s, so we'll never be able to find out if he was the transmitter, but he probably was, since my mother is in her 90s and going strong.

"I always thought it was better to live with denial and the assumption that everything would be fine. That's why I never mentioned this to my son, Robert. If you figure the odds, my chances are 50/50. Robert has a 25-percent chance, and his children only have a 12.5-percent chance—pretty small—so I've just kept it to myself.

"Yes, I've been worried about my brother Charles. I hoped it was Parkinsonism, but it did begin to look like what I remember of Mary. There's nothing you can do about Huntington's, so what would have been the point of telling him my suspicions? I'm not sure there's any point even now. If you could treat it, that would be a different matter.

"As for me, the last 25 years since Mary died have been good ones. I've watched Robert grow up and become successful. My wife and I have been happily married, my law practice has done better than I deserved, and I've had time to be active in civic organizations. Do you think I could have done better if I knew that I wouldn't come down with Huntington's disease? Would it have been better if I knew I would get it when I was 40, or 50, or 60? I doubt it. It would have been a terrible burden to bear. Granted, I could have encouraged Robert not to have children by his first wife. He might even have listened, but then he would not have had the pleasure of watching them grow up. And he would have had to carry that burden, too, for even longer than I.

"I appreciate your concern, Dr. Gunderson. Thanks for listening to me. I guess I've kept it bottled up too long—you can tell—but it was better that way and I still think it is. Of course, you'll be keeping this information confidential, just between the two of us. As for Virginia, I don't care what that dame wants. If she's so desperate for a perfect baby, let her go adopt one or something. She's not my problem. The rest of the family is and I'd just as soon leave things the way they've been. If Charles has Huntington's, it will all come out soon enough."

Mr. Smyth's Dilemma

What do you think about Mr. Smyth's position? Is living with denial a reasonable approach to a problem such as Huntington's? What are the consequences of such an approach for him and for his family?

Would he have been better if he had assumed the glass was half empty and acted as if he would come down with the disease? He could have increased his insurance, set his affairs in order, and taken a stable job with good benefits. Would this have been wise?

Should he have told his brother Charles? Did Charles have the right to know so he could make his own plans? Now that Charles is showing manifestations of the disease, should he be told? Will it help Charles or his wife? What about Charles' children, would they have decided not to have children of their own?

How about Robert and his children?

What would you have done if you had been in Mr. Smyth's shoes 20 to 25 years ago? What would you do if you were in his shoes now? Remember, Charles' disease will probably be diagnosed soon.

Do these individuals have the right to know their risk for Huntington's disease? Do they have the right *not* to know? How would they exercise either of these rights when they did not even know they were at risk for Huntington's disease?

Did Mr. Smyth have a duty to tell the others about Mary's condition and their own risks? What is the source of that duty? How would you resolve the conflicts between the rights of those who would want to know and of those who would not want to know without first telling them about Mary? If you tell them about Mary then they know they are at risk.

Try analyzing these issues with the utilitarian approach of the greatest happiness for the greatest number. What would have been the benefits of Mr. Smyth having told the family about Mary's disease 25 years ago? Would Charles have been happier knowing of his 50-percent risk? How about his children, who will soon learn of their own risk? How about Robert? Would he have had children in his previous marriage had he known?

Using this analysis, what should Mr. Smyth have done 25 years ago? What should he do now?

Now redo your analysis using a Kantian approach of rights and duties to answer the same questions. Do these two moral analyses yield the same results?

Dr. Gunderson's Dilemma

"Dr. Gunderson, it's a counselor from the Pregnancy Counseling Center on the phone asking to speak with you about Charles Smyth. Would you like me to pull his chart?"

"No, thank you. Dr. Gunderson speaking. Yes, I take care of him. Can you tell me what this is about?"

"I'm a counselor at the Genetics Center and I have a patient who has come to us for genetic counseling. She is engaged to Robert Smyth. We were told that his Uncle Charles, who is under your care, has a neurological disorder, and we are checking to be sure it isn't any genetic disease that we should know about. I always like to be sure I'm accurate when I provide counseling."

"Hello . . . are you still there, Dr. Gunderson?"

Put yourself in Dr. Gunderson's position. What will you respond? You have only a few seconds before the pause will become embarrassing. If you think quickly you could tell her that you have to get the patient's chart and will call her back. That could give you time to think.

Should you tell her the truth? If you don't, she won't be telling the truth to Virginia. A baby may result that could have Huntington's disease 50 years from now. What is the truth? Do you know as a fact that Charles has Huntington's? Do you merely suspect it? What effect does yesterday's disclosure about Charles' sister have on the level of your suspicion? It should increase it appreciably, but the diagnosis is still not certain.

How does the fact that Mr. Smyth asked you to keep the information about Mary confidential bear on your decision? Should you tell the truth (whatever it may be) to this counselor when you have not yet told Charles and his wife?

Does Virginia, who is not your patient nor even a member of the family, have any right to know?

Outline your justification for what you will tell the counselor: the truth? part truth? a lie? an evasion? Could you tell her your dilemma and pledge her to keep it confidential, thus putting her in your situation. Would her situation be different since Virginia *is* her patient?

Charles' Response

"Thanks for telling me, Henry," Charles replies glumly when his brother finally tells him. "You know, I don't remember much about Mary. I was younger and it was kept very quiet. I always thought Mom was embarrassed about having her in a mental institution. But I remember some of the whispers, and Mom going out to visit her. I think I've suspected this past year that I might have the same thing, but I was afraid to find out. In a way it's a comfort to know what I've got. At least now I know how to plan.

"And thanks for not burdening me with this information over all these years. It must have been a terrible responsibility for you to make that decision and to keep the secret, but it certainly made my life easier.

"I guess I'll have to tell my kids now. I hope they'll be able to cope.

I guess their biggest decision will be whether or not to have children of their own. If I've got Huntington's, then they each have a 50-percent chance, and their children will have a 25-percent chance? Is that right? Or will my grandchildren's chances each be either 50 percent or zero, with nothing in between. I wish there were a test for the disease. It would be a great relief if they could know that they would be okay . . . but what if they found out that they would come down with it 20 or 30 or 40 years from now?

"Anyway, you're a wonderful older brother. Thanks."

* * *

If there were Huntington's in your family and there were a safe, reliable test, would you want to know if you were affected or only if you were unaffected? You cannot know one without the other. Would you have children, knowing their chances of the disease?

Virginia's Response

"That bastard! Robert, do you realize what he's done to you and almost done to me! If you have that terrible disease you could become an invalid, a vegetable, or worse, a moving vegetable, in 10 years. He allowed you to have children without even knowing, without being able to make an informed decision! They could have it, too! What right did he have to keep it all to himself? Who does he think he is, God? You had the right to make your own decisions.

"Poor Robert. I hope you don't get it. I don't know if I could stand watching you deteriorate. I am not the kind who could feed you and bathe you and treat you like an infant. Robert, what are we going to do?"

* * *

Is Virginia's response unreasonable? How would you have responded if you suddenly found that your fiancé had a 50-percent chance of a progressive, crippling, dementing disease? Would you go through with marriage? Would you have children if they could be affected? If there were Huntington's in your fiancé's family, would you want your fiancé tested (if there was a test)? Would your marriage depend on your fiancé's having the test? What would you do if it were positive? Do you have the right to require your fiancé to bear or potentially bear this tremendous burden? Does he (or she) have the right to refuse? If a test were available (and it will be shortly), what are his or her obligations to you? To prospective children? Do information and truth make such decisions easier or more difficult?

A genetic test for Huntington's disease is almost ready for use. Think about the guidelines you would prepare for using this test when it becomes available. Who should be able to request it? Who will receive the results? How will you protect those who don't want to know? How will you assure the rights of spouses, fiancés, children, and prospective children? What ethical theory will you use to justify your guidelines?

Chapter 11

Baby James

"You want to do what? You want to kill a perfectly healthy young baboon, take its heart, and transplant it into a sickly kid? What about the baboon?" shouts Mr. Smith. "That's nothing but pure speciesism!" George Smith represents the Animal Rights League on South General Hospital's Institutional Review Board, a committee that reviews all medical experiments done at the hospital. You've heard his outraged explosions before, but this does sound like a crazy idea.

But Dr. H. Baldwin Spence remains his usual calm, aloof self. "It's the baby's only chance for survival. Would you rather he died than that ape? Besides, they already tried such a transplant in California and it was successful, at least for a while. That procedure put their hospital on the map, and the surgeon too. This is South General's chance to be famous. I've been working on transplanting hearts, livers, and kidneys from one species to another for 4 years now. It turns out to be easy if you have the size right, and that baboon's heart is just about the right size for the baby. It shouldn't be any problem."

"Just a minute, Baldwin," you say. "As chairman of this Research Review Board, I have a responsibility to run it and to do things in a logical order. I know you're pressed for time and you haven't filed a written application, but start at the beginning and tell us about the child and the research you're proposing."

"It's not research," says Dr. Spence. "We're not experimenting with this child, we're trying therapy, innovative therapy. It's his only hope. I'm not even sure why I decided to present this to you, since we try new things in the operating room all the time. But, because this operation will generate a lot of press, I thought you should know about it. I don't need your approval, but it would be nice to have your support. We're planning to do the operation first thing tomorrow morning if we have the parents' permission.

115

"Baby James was born with a severe abnormality of the heart. He has terrible trouble breathing because of all the blood and fluid backed up in his lungs. He's in heart failure and, despite all the medication to get rid of fluid and strengthen the heart, he's getting worse. We've only seen one baby like him, and that baby died in two weeks. There are a number of these babies reported in the literature, and many things have been tried. None of them work. At the last Academy meeting some hotshot at one of those Boston hospitals said he had a new surgical approach, but only two of the five babies were alive six months after the operation. So there's really no alternative. If we put in this baboon's heart, who knows?"

Dr. H. Baldwin Spence is impressive. You know he trained as a cardiac surgeon at Boston Metropolitan and then came back home. He is the best (and richest) cardiac surgeon in the area and a community leader as well. He used his own money and his family's money to set up the Spence Cardiac Research Lab, where he worked on his transplants. Maybe he's right. Why not try it? What's there to lose? Just trying it would show that South General was no backwater hospital. If they can do something like that, it might even increase referrals and help to keep the hospital's beds filled.

"What about informed consent?" you ask. "What have you told the parents?"

"What do you mean? What are you insinuating? I told them the absolute truth; I always tell patients the truth! I told them that the baby has a bad abnormality of the heart. That's he's in heart failure and is going to die soon, like all the other babies with this problem. I told them that we've been working with animal transplants and have put dog hearts into pigs and goat hearts into dogs. There would be no special trick to putting a baboon's heart into their baby. It's the same size and almost the same genetically. Besides, there's nothing else to do except to let him die. The parents are simple country folk, but they understood. They didn't even have any questions. They just said okay. However, I wanted them to go back and think about it some more while we got things together for the operation. They're coming back this evening, and we plan to talk again before tomorrow's operation."

South General Hospital is not on the transplant frontier. We have done some kidney transplants, but never hearts or other organs, so the committee does not have much expertise in this area.

"Any questions?" you ask of the other members.

"What if it doesn't work?" asks Dr. Pebbles, the pediatrician on the committee.

"Well, the baby will be no worse off than if we hadn't done it," replies Dr. Spence. "I guess he dies."

"Why not use a human heart transplant?" asks Dr. Brink from internal medicine.

"You know how hard it is to get donors, even for adults, even when you have days and weeks to look. We're planning this operation for tomorrow, and I'm not aware of any donors. We're continuing to look, but I don't expect to be successful."

"Any more questions? If not, thank you, Dr. Spence. We'd like to chat a bit among ourselves, and we'll be in touch with you this afternoon."

"I suggest transplanting the heart of that arrogant, stupid, stuffed-shirt playboy into the baby and save the life of the baboon in the process. But his heart's probably not big enough to sustain the baby. Just big enough to support his pea-sized brain," roars Mr. Smith. "You only have to follow the newspapers and television to know that pigs, goats, and sheep are genetically different from one another, and they are all different from humans. Transplants are more than just plumbing. Sure you can transplant a pig's heart into a goat; it fits, but it won't work for long because of tissue rejection. Spence doesn't understand rejection; he may think it has to do with blackballs and country clubs. Think of all of the sheep, goats, and pigs he's wasted. It's immoral!"

"Sometimes even you say sensible things," interrupts Dr. Pebbles. "I know a fair bit about immunology from the allergy work I do with kids. I know enough to know Baldwin's deficiencies, and that transplant immunology is not strong here at South General. Even if he gets away with the technical problems of transplanting the heart, he's not equipped to handle the problems of immunosuppression or even detecting transplant rejection. Has he even done tissue typing? He didn't mention it."

"Would a human infant heart be better, if one could be found?" asked Reverend Tolson.

"Who knows? You still have the immunologic problems, maybe less than between species. He's counting on the fact that a young infant won't make sufficient antibodies to reject the transplant. I don't see how we can let him barge ahead. He doesn't understand what he's doing."

"Oh, yes, he does," says Smith. "He's trying to make a name for himself like Christian Barnard. Spence wants to be the first to do something. He's not interested in the infant or the baboon.

"Couldn't we send this infant somewhere else? To Boston or Johns Hopkins?"

"That's not our job, George. It's Spence's patient. Our job is to assure the ethics of the research."

"Then we have a problem," interjects Dr. Brink. "Spence says it isn't research. He specifically called it 'innovative therapy,' and if he's right he didn't have to come to us for approval. When a physician or a surgeon does something for a patient's benefit, that's solely between the doctor and the patient. If I want to use a drug available for the treatment of asthma to treat a patient's cancer, that's my right. I should explain it to my patient and get his permission. If his toes drop off during treatment, he can sue me. That's my problem. Only if I plan to ask questions, learn something, or do a study does it become research, and research requires this committee's approval. That's how surgeons get away with all that they do in the operating room without coming to the committee. They just say, 'Today we're going to put the lungs in backward and see if the patient breathes better.' If the patient survives, they write a paper on 'Pulmonary Inversion and the Cure of Flatulence,' or some such thing."

"I think we're getting off track here. I believe I detect some animosity to surgeons. Dr. Pebbles, your turn."

"I don't trust this fellow any more than you do, but our alternative seems to be to let this little tyke die. Does that accomplish anything? There isn't much time for this infant. He'll die in the next couple of days. Could we compromise and let Spence do the operation on the condition that it's only a temporizing procedure until a human infant heart is found? Then the baby could be transferred to a transplantation center for the final transplant and the immunologic management. That way, Spence could be the first and the baby could get good care—if a center would take him."

"We could get some good public relations out of it, too," murmurs the vice president of the hospital, who now seems interested in the discussion.

"Let's step back for a minute," you say, "and look at the role of this committee. Is it our job merely to review research on humans to be sure that it is ethical? If so, we have to answer the question of whether this is even research. If our role is broader, we have to ask if this is good or at least morally acceptable practice. How would we have known about this planned operation ahead of time if Spence hadn't come to us? Will people stop coming to the committee if we say no? Should we just say that this isn't our province and let Spence do his thing? Should we say no, you can't do the operation? If so, do we have the authority to enforce a decision? Would that help the baby, or just save us bad publicity? Should we intervene as Dr. Pebbles' suggested and find a center to take over?

"We've got to decide what the role of this committee should be. A hospital like this doesn't have the personnel to afford a separate ethics committee like big hospitals have."

* * *

As chairman of the committee, how would you resolve the multiple issues raised? For example:

1. Is this research, or just innovative therapy? Does Spence need your permission? If not, what role should the committee play? Would it be ethical for the committee *not* to play a role?
2. Did the parents give informed consent? Did Dr. Spence present fair and unbiased information? Could he have, when this type of operation has not been done before? Were alternatives and consequences presented or considered? Do the parents really understand? Could "simple folk" understand the multiple problems involved? Were they given a choice they couldn't refuse? Even if the parents were experts in biology and gave truly informed consent, is it moral to do the operation?
3. What are the obligations to try something new that might work, when there is no standard therapy that would be effective? Is it better just to stand there than to do something?
4. Is this procedure being done for the infant's benefit? Is it being done to benefit other infants? Or for Dr. Spence's benefit? Does it matter? How do you tell? When benefits are in conflict, how do you resolve the differences? Does the potential good or bad publicity pose a conflict for the hospital?
5. Would the operation be a "benefit" to Baby James by giving meaning to his life even if it were a failure? What would the benefit be to him of not doing it and allowing him to die?
6. Is there any merit to the arguments of the animal rights groups that removal of the heart from an animal for the benefit of a human is "speciesism" and that animals also have rights?

Now that you have carefully considered these issues: (1) vote to approve permission for the operation; (2) vote to refuse permission for the operation; (3) vote that this is not research and does not require approval from this committee; (4) vote for some other option.
Defend the moral basis for your vote.

Chapter 12

The Castelli Baby

"It's cruel and inhumane! You people must be sadists, torturing little children. Do you do it just for the challenge? Don't you ever think of those poor kids and what it must be like? You treat them like objects, not like babies!"

As Rachel's tirade ends, Bernstein thinks, "That's the last time I tell my wife about a case at the dinner table. It's been a tough day. Up all last night struggling with this newborn, finally get home for a little peace and quiet, and now this. Damn! No one appreciates what you do. First, that soft-headed intern asking all those ethical questions when I was busy teaching him how to save the infant's life. Then the attending trying to enliven rounds with questions about 'what is a person' and all this garbage about rights, duties, and other theoretical junk when he should have been teaching about things like fluids and urinary output. These interns would be hard put to save lives with all that ethical stuff.

"Getting to sleep isn't easy. It never is when you've been going 90 miles per hour for 36 hours straight. It's hard work being a fellow in neonatology at University Hospital—especially when you're in charge of the intensive care nursery. Those 40 babies all depend on you. The interns don't know much, especially this time of year. You have to check everything, tell them what to do, and then watch that they do it right. This is why you've gone into medicine—to care for children and to teach. If you let interns do something wrong, the baby dies. If you make sure they do it right, the child lives. Even the assistant residents, who are supposed to be in charge, don't have a lot of experience and they require supervision.

"The Castelli baby, last night's sleep buster, is a good example. He was born about 6 P.M. by Caesarian section because of fetal distress. They called ahead of time. The mother is 32, a professional of some sort. The infant was born blue and not breathing, limp. It was a chance to show the new intern how to intubate and breathe for the baby. Even with all the attention, it was twenty minutes before the baby could breathe on his own, and he still needed assistance. Clearly, the infant was severely hypoxic.

"As expected, the baby had crisis after crisis all night long, and it was an opportunity to teach the resident and students how to deal with each one—a great teaching case. Seizures during the first few hours—they learned how to use anticonvulsants and later how to hold back fluids, anticipating the effect of the lack of oxygen on the kidneys, heart, and liver. Medication to support his blood pressure, digitalis for the heart. It was right out of a textbook. The student and intern were lucky to have me to teach them and to have cases like that to learn from. It was really great teaching material and it was handled magnificently."

You are the assistant resident in the nursery. In the morning you start rounds at 7:30 with Dr. Bernstein and the team of interns and students. They bring you up to date on the babies in the nursery. The 1½-pound infant is doing well, his intracranial hemorrhage resolving. The twins seem to be growing and should be out in three to four weeks. The baby with esophageal atresia is doing as well as can be expected after surgery. There are only two cases that are likely to die—the new premature with massive intraventricular hemorrhage and the one with the pneumonia and lung disase.

You tell the troops, "It looks like a quiet day except for the Castelli infant admitted Monday night. He's now 36-hours-old."

When the Castelli name is mentioned, Bernstein's face lights up. "He's a fascinating case with lots of pathology. A good lesson about all the problems of severe hypoxia and its effects on the nervous system. Let's discuss him in the lounge over coffee."

"Rick," Bernstein quizzes the medical student, "tell the group what you learned about seizures in the newborn from those references I gave you yesterday."

"Seizures in the newborn have many causes, but when they start in the first hours of life they are usually due to lack of oxygen to the brain. The earlier they start and the harder to control, the worse the brain damage has been and the worse the outlook. In this case, the infant was blue and limp at birth, so you knew he had been hypoxic. Seizures started in the first hours of life and didn't respond to phenobarbital or to the other anticonvulsant medications we've used—phenytoin and paraldehyde—so we have good evidence that the hypoxia was severe. One article cited statistics; one third of those infants died. Of the babies like this who survived, 80 percent were significantly retarded with cerebral palsy."

"Good job, Rick. Karen, what other problems are related to hypoxia?"

"Depending on its severity and duration, they can be multiple. You may see evidence of heart failure, and we've seen some of this in Castelli. You can use diuretics to get rid of the excess fluid, but it's a problem because the kidneys often shut down, as this baby's have. So you have to watch the fluids very carefully. Digitalis helps with the arrythmias and strengthens the heart. They get liver failure as well and this can cause problems particularly with bilirubin. If the infant survives, most of these problems go away."

"What about the bowel, Karen?"

"These babies can get what's called necrotizing enterocolitis in which the bowel dies from lack of blood supply. This becomes obvious about the third to fourth day—if it occurs."

"Good. Let's talk some about acid-base problems. You've got this baby whose pH is 7.1, his CO_2 is. . . ."

Teaching rounds are supposed to begin at 11 A.M. sharp, but Dr. Kendrick is rarely on time. He's one of the more casual faculty; perhaps it goes back to his days as a practicing pediatrician before he joined the faculty at University. He prides himself on being one of University's few full-time clinicians, not one of those "lab types." He talks a lot about the art of medicine. Castelli is the most complicated case and the logical one to present on teaching rounds.

The intern presents the case. The blood gases and chemistries are neatly tallied on the board. Bernstein is very proud of how the case has been managed so far, and the intern did a good job of presenting the facts.

Dr. Kendrick nods. "Nice job, guys. Now, tell me about the family. What are they like? What do they think about all this? What have you told them?"

"The student spoke with the father yesterday," you reply. "He told them that the baby was very sick and might not make it, but we were doing everything possible. I haven't had time to meet them yet."

"What do they do? Does the mother work? Do they have other children? Have you told them the outlook for this child if he survives—the high chance of cerebral palsy and mental retardation? Have you asked them what they want you to do, how far you should go?"

Mary, Castelli's primary nurse, finally broke the embarrassing silence. "I spoke to Mrs. Castelli yesterday afternoon. She was pretty depressed and tearful. She's a writer for one of the major women's magazines. She's read a lot of the stories about babies like this and about the families' reactions to them—maybe she's written some. I think she understands the baby's problems. She's 32 and they've waited a long time for this child—until they had a house and were settled into their careers. Mr.

Castelli is an engineer for the utility company. I don't know if Mrs. Castelli was crying for the baby or for herself. She's afraid that all their future plans are ruined."

"Thank you, Mary," says Dr. Kendrick. "At least someone in this room is concerned about more than the baby's chemistries."

"I spent thirty-six hours saving this kid's life!" Bernstein responds. "We've controlled the seizures, taken care of his heart failure, and managed his fluids. Look at those chemistries—he's in good shape. What more do you want us to do?"

"Have you ever thought about what you shouldn't do?" Kendrick then turns to Rick, the medical student. "Rick, what do you think life would be like if you had a child who was profoundly retarded with cerebral palsy? A child who responded, smiled, maybe made his needs known, but who couldn't get around without braces, crutches, and your constant help? What will it be like for the Castellis? Will Mrs. Castelli be able to continue her career? Will Mr. Castelli be able to take risks, such as changing jobs? It certainly won't be the life they planned. Should they have any say in what you're doing for the baby?"

"I don't know," responds Rick. "I haven't had any experience like that. But when I talked with my girlfriend about what I've seen in the nursery this month, I'm not sure we want children. I don't know if we could handle the risk of a baby like the one you describe. But isn't our job as physicians to look out for the baby? If a couple decides to have a child, don't they also take on an obligation to care for that child if it's damaged? Isn't that one of the risks of becoming a parent?"

"That's a very important point," smiled Kendrick approvingly, "but this isn't just a tragedy for the parents. Look at it from the child's viewpoint. What would such a life be like? Would it be a life worth living?"

"Would you rather that Castelli was dead?" exclaimed the intern. "I'm sure that the family would rather that the baby and his problems would just go away, but that's not possible. We haven't done anything heroic or extraordinary or any of those terms that ethicists use. We've just done the standard things we do every day in this nursery. Castelli just required more of them."

"Did you have permission to do them? Did the family give informed consent?" asks Kendrick.

"We don't get informed consent for everything we do down here," Bernstein replies. "There's too much to do. We'd be spending all our time explaining and talking while the babies died. I don't think more than the general consent form we use for every baby in the nursery is required for ordinary care."

"That raises a very interesting set of questions that we should talk about at length on one of these rounds," says Kendrick, "but we're short of time now." Kendrick then turns to you and says, "Unless you want Bernstein to run everything down here, you'd better get to know the Castellis and talk with them about the baby. One never knows when an infant like this is going to require something heroic as an emergency. Then you really would need their permission, an informed permission, and might not have time to obtain it."

* * *

Your meeting with the Castellis that afternoon went well. They are very nice, intelligent people, and they obviously care about the baby. You review the problems to date, and they are very appreciative of the care the whole staff is giving to Chris; Christopher is the name they have chosen. They particularly mention Mary, Chris's Primary Nurse,—their conversations with her have been reassuring. When you talk about the baby's outlook, things get rougher. They are very anxious about what life will be like for Chris if he is severely retarded and has cerebral palsy; an 80-percent chance of brain damage is not good odds, but there is hope. You reassure them that you are not doing anything painful or heroic, and with luck Chris will come off the ventilator in a few days. You felt you had to tell them about possible future complications. Then it hits the fan. You mention the possibilities of rupture of the lung, intracranial bleeding, and the breakdown of the bowel. It is not clear which one does it, but at this point Mr. Castelli becomes adamant.

"Look," he says, "the baby has gone through enough! His chances for any kind of a reasonable life are small. You can't just torture and experiment on him for nothing. He's a human being, for God's sake! If any of those things happens and decreases his chances even further, then I'm not sure it's worth it!"

You reassure Mr. Castelli that before doing anything major, the parents' permission is required. You also tell the Castellis that they are welcome to see the baby any time and that you will keep them informed.

At 1 A.M. Thursday the intern calls. Chris Castelli has suddenly turned sour. You rush from the sleeping quarters to find a blue baby with a pulse of 170. A quick listen to the chest reveals no breath sounds on the left side.

"He's ruptured his lung," you mumble aloud, "pneumothorax—not an uncommon problem for these infants on respirators. No time for a chest X-ray. Get me a twenty-gauge needle and a large syringe," you call.

The needle in the chest is both diagnostic and therapeutic. Once the air that had been compressing the lung was removed, Chris turns pinker and his heartbeat returns to normal.

"Good work picking that up quickly," you tell the intern. "Now we have to get the surgeon to put in a chest tube so the air doesn't reaccumulate. Check with the operator to see who's on call."

"Don't we have to get an operation permit for that?" asks the nurse.

"Yes, I guess we do. I promised to keep the parents informed, anyway. I'll call Mr. Castelli."

Mr. Castelli's response to your request is a decided "No! I told you this afternoon that we didn't want anything heroic done and I haven't changed my mind. It's not in the baby's best interest. I didn't even give you permission to put that needle in his chest, did I?"

Your efforts to persuade Mr. Castelli are most frustrating. "Placing a chest tube is not heroic; it's done all the time in the nursery. It doesn't require anesthesia, just a little local numbing. The tube will only be in for a few days, then the lung will heal itself. If we don't do it the air may reaccumulate and the baby will die. The outlook for mental retardation or cerebral palsy hasn't changed. They're no worse than they were this afternoon."

Hearing all this, Bernstein picks up the phone, and it is his argument that is finally successful.

"Look, Mr. Castelli," he says, "if we don't do this simple operation your baby will die. The operation has to be done! Either you give permission for it, or I'll just do it as an emergency and get a court order in the morning and assume medical custody of the child. The surgeon is here now. Which way do you want it?"

Given that choice, Mr. Castelli caves in. "But this is all," he says. "You are *not* to do any more surgery or anything else heroic without specific written permission. I will send a notarized letter to that effect in the morning!"

The chest tube is inserted uneventfully.

On rounds that morning, Dr. Kendrick returns to the subject of the Castelli baby. "Would you really have gone to court if they didn't give permission? Didn't you assault the baby by inserting the needle without their permison? Are you confident you could justify that as emergency treatment? How would you justify the placement of a chest catheter to prevent future problems if Mr. Castelli hadn't given in? Does your role as the baby's physician give you the right to do what you think best for the baby? Or is that right still the parent's prerogative?"

More rhetorical questions, but you have to admit that Dr. Kendrick has given you and the staff a lot to think about.

Bernstein explodes. "Dr. Kendrick, I'm up to my ears with all these ethical questions. I am sick and tired of being second-guessed on rounds the morning after. When you are willing to get out of your warm bed at

1 A.M. and come into the nursery and care for the sick infants and make these decisions yourself, then perhaps we can talk about ethics.

"You didn't treat the low pH! You didn't treat the child's kidney failure! You didn't try and stop his seizures! And you weren't here last night when he was blue and couldn't breathe. You can talk all you like, but I wasn't about to let this baby die when I could do something simple with a needle. What's more, I wasn't about to let it happen again; that's why the chest tube was inserted.

"This is my patient, and I'm going to give him the best care I know how. I feel sorry for his parents, and I'll help them as best I can, but they are not my patients, the baby is! He comes first! All the things you are talking about—prerogatives, parent's rights and feelings—these are all secondary questions. Patient care has to come first!"

Bernstein storms out of the room.

* * *

Pause here and think about those questions. What do you think about Bernstein as a person? As a physician? Would you like to be his kind of physician? Do you find him arrogant? Mechanical? Insensitive? Do you think he likes his role of saving sick infants from death? Is this playing God? Does he give adequate consideration to the parents? Is he sufficiently sensitive to the child and his future problems?

What do you think about Dr. Kendrick as a physician? Would you rather have him as your doctor? Would he be a better role model? Is he more caring, sensitive, and empathetic? Is he as competent, medically aggressive, and effective? Whose critically ill patients are more likely to survive?

How would you choose between bedside manner and aggressive competence? Which doctor would you prefer for your child?

What moral considerations would you have used en route to the nursery at 1 A.M.? Would or should you have considered parental rights and appropriate consent when faced with the baby who was blue? What decision-making process should Bernstein or Kendrick have gone through at that time?

* * *

The real zinger comes at the end of these rounds when the ultrasound technician brings in the study she has just performed on Chris. There is evidence of a massive intracranial hemorrhage—something doubtlessly caused by the pneumothorax and the increased venous pressure that it produced. Now the outlook for the baby is even worse. His 20-percent chance for a normal outcome has diminished considerably.

126

"Well?" Dr. Kendrick asks. "What are you going to do now? I suppose you could take him off the respirator. If you offer the parents that alternative, I think they might jump at it. If you don't offer it, they may request it themselves. They're pretty sophisticated. You could go on meeting each crisis as it occurs, but there's a substantial chance that tomorrow or the next day he'll show evidence of bowel infarction; then you'll either have to let him go or fight the parents to allow an operation to remove the dead bowel. And it's too early to tell but, with the oxygen he requires, he could become blind from retrolental fibroplasia. You better plan ahead and avoid a recurrence of these 1 A.M. crises."

There is a lively discussion among the staff. Some feel that the baby has suffered enough and you should turn off the respirator. Others feel that you couldn't do this because the baby isn't brain dead; there are no criteria for brain death in infants, anyway. Several people feel that this is the parents' decision. Others feel that their decision would be too self-serving, and it is the physician's job to be the child's advocate. There clearly is no consensus about what to advocate.

Since you are the baby's physician, what will you do now? It seems that there are several options.

1. You could decide to quit, turn off the respirator, and let Chris die. It would be the quickest way out of this mess. You would, of course, have to talk with the Castellis and get their agreement, but they would probably be eager to agree. If you choose this option, outline the main points of the discussion you would have with them and justify your decision. Why is it so different from your discussion when you put in the chest tube last night? Then turn to the next section, "You Decide to Quit" (p. 128).

2. You could continue treating Chris as you have been, handling each crisis if and when it occurs. Be aware that many of these sick prematures develop many problems. He could get pneumonia; would you treat that with antibiotics? He could get hydrocephalus (water on the brain); would you put in a shunt, a tube to drain the fluid into the abdomen where it will be absorbed? It's not a big operation. The shunt could get infected or blocked; would you fix it? He could get bowel infarction, requiring the removal of most of his intestine and continued feeding by vein for years; would that treatment be too much? Is there a point at which you would decide that you had done enough? Where is that point? How would you determine it? If you choose this option, turn to "You Continue Treating Chris" (p. 129).

127

3. You could decide that this ethical stuff is getting just too complicated and you need some help. If so, perhaps you should turn to the hospital's Infant Care Review Committee for consultation. If you choose this course, turn to "The Infant Care Review Committee" (p. 129).

You Decide to Quit

Your discussion with the Castellis goes well. With the additional information about the intracerebral hemorrhage and its further effects on Chris's chances for a reasonable life, they readily agree that the future quality of life for Chris would be so bad that he would be better off dead. They are very appreciative of your willingness to relieve his burden.

You go back to the nursery and explain your plan to the team. Priscilla, the assistant head nurse, has a very different idea.

"Doctor," she says, "you can't do that, not in my nursery! You are just bending to what these yuppie parents want for themselves. There are very specific rules that you have to follow—and what you are proposing is clearly medical neglect. You cannot say that this baby is chronically and irreversibly comatose or that your treatment is futile, and what you or the parents think about quality of future life isn't pertinent. If you turn off the respirator, you'll be breaking the law."

* * *

Do you want to reconsider your plan in light of Priscilla's vehemence? If so, go back and choose again. If not, read the next section.

If you think you need some additional help and thought, consult with the Infant Care Review Committee. Turn to the section entitled "The Infant Care Review Committee" (p. 129).

You Turn Off the Respirator

Four days ago you turned off the respirator and declared Chris dead. Priscilla called the Child Abuse Agency, which contacted the chairman of the hospital's Infant Care Review Committee. He told them that he knew nothing about the case, but would collaborate with the Child Abuse Agency's investigation of the charge of medical neglect. The hospital lawyer called you in and told you that as far as he could see, you clearly had not met the criteria of the Baby Doe regulations. There is no telling what the Child Abuse Agency would do, since this is the first solid case that has come before them. If they find that this was medical neglect, they will turn it over to the district attorney for whatever action he feels appropriate.

The phone calls from the press really get to you. They are calling from all over, ever since the local paper published the article headlined, "Physician Pulls The Plug: Child Abuse Team Investigating."

The head of the ICRC asks you to prepare a written statement justifying your action and your avoidance of his committee. He specifically encourages you to review form 3A (p. 130) and respond in detail to each of the items.

When you have completed this task, read the section entitled "The Infant Care Review Committee Meets" (p. 131).

You Continue Treating Chris

It's three days later, and Castelli continues to be "a textbook case." His kidneys have not started working. Today he shows the evidence of infarction of the bowel and, what is more, the ultrasound shows enlargement of the ventricles within the brain. He is developing hydrocephalus from the hemorrhage. It seems you have been fighting a losing battle. Whatever you do would seem futile.

Further discussion on rounds leads you to turn to the Infant Care Review Committee for affirmation before you turn off the respirator.

The Infant Care Review Committee

You speak to the secretary of the Infant Care Review Committee. The committee would be pleased to meet with you and to review the problem. She will call the committee together tomorrow afternoon. In the meantime, would you please fill out ICRC form 3A, which she will bring to you.

ICRC form 3A appears below. Please fill it out completely and fill in the section labeled "Action of the Committee" with your impression of their anticipated response.

Form 3A

University Hospital Infant Care Review Committee

In preparation for our meetings, we have found it useful to have the petitioner be aware of the Child Abuse and Neglect Prevention and Treatment Program established by the U.S. Department of Health and Human Services. Its regulations define medical neglect. "Medical neglect means failure to respond to an infant's life-threatening condition by providing treatment that, in the treating physician's reasonable medical judgment, will be most likely to be effective in ameliorating or correcting all such conditions."

Exceptions may be made when:

1. The infant is chronically or irreversibly comatose.
2. Such treatment would merely prolong dying or not be effective in ameliorating or correcting all the infant's life-threatening conditions or otherwise be futile in terms of survival of the infant.
3. Such treatment would be virtually futile in terms of the survival of the infant and the treatment itself under such circumstances would be inhumane.

Please respond to these questions in writing as completely as possible.

1. State the question you are asking the committee (please be succinct).

2. Are you proposing something that could be construed as medical neglect by you or others (see above)?

3. Is the infant chronically and irreversibly comatose (Yes/No)?

4. Would the proposed treatment:
   (a) "Merely prolong dying?" Explain.

(b) "Not be effective in correcting or ameliorating all life threatening conditions?" Explain.

(c) "Be otherwise futile in terms of survival of the infant?" Explain.

5. Would the proposed treatment be:
   (a) "Virtually futile in terms of survival of the infant?" Explain.

   (b) "And Inhumane?" Explain.

6. Are there other special factors that the committee should consider?
   Explain.

Response of the committee (may be continued on separate page).

This form is based on the regulations that implement the Child Abuse
Amendments of 1984 published in the *Federal Register,* April 15, 1985,
Part 1340, pp. 14887–888.

When you have completed this form, turn to the next section.

The Infant Care Review Committee Meets

"Gentlemen and ladies," Dr. Orville Gross begins. "We have before us today the case of Christopher Castelli, a newborn with multiple problems.
The issue is whether and when to stop treatment. First, we might approach
this by reviewing form 3A, which we have before us. If this infant meets
the criteria of the published regulations, then withholding or stopping
treatment will not be medical neglect.

"Is this infant 'chronically and irreversibly comatose?' You indicate
that there is no way of telling in a sick infant of this age."

"Would the treatment 'merely prolong dying?' You state on the form that the infant is not dying now, but he has severe brain damage and in all likelihood would have profound mental retardation and cerebral palsy. Do you have anything to add? Has anything changed since you filled out the forms?"

"No, sir," you respond. "Nothing has changed in the past twenty-four hours. We anticipate that the baby is likely to have infarction of the bowel, which will show itself in the next few days. This would require major surgery to remove part of the bowel, and there might not be enough left for him to get adequate nutrition. He also has a good chance of developing hydrocephalus from his intracranial bleed and. . . ."

"Thank you. We are dealing with the baby's current condition. Later, if you want, we can deal with the possible future problems.

"You propose to turn off the respirator. Is it 'effective in correcting or ameliorating all the infant's life-threatening conditions? Or otherwise futile in terms of survival of the infant?' Clearly not, since you state the infant currently has no life-threatening conditions. Similarly, the treatment is neither 'virtually futile nor inhumane,' is it? At this time you are only providing the ordinary care that you give to many babies in your nursery."

"Well, sir," you reply, "it could be considered inhumane to keep a baby like this on a respirator."

"That's not the issue. The treatment has to be *both* virtually futile (which it is not) and inhumane.

"As I see it, this poor, unfortunate child does not meet the criteria of the regulations. Despite the empathy and sympathy that I am sure we all feel for the baby and the family, I don't see how we could sanction turning off the respirator."

* * *

What do you think? Is the chairman correct in stating that discontinuing the respirator at this time would be "medical neglect" as defined in the regulations? If you were a member of the committee, would you vote to allow it? Or would you reject the request? Please defend whichever position you take. Then continue reading.

The Meeting of the Infant Care
Review Committee Continues

"Dr. Gross, I strongly object to your absolutely literal interpretation of the regulations," begins Dr. Kendrick. "Even the Department of Health and Human Services requires many pages to explain what they think the words mean. The key words in the regulations are, I believe, 'in the opinion of a reasonable physician.' I am a 'reasonable physician' familiar with this case. I believe that this child is irreversibly comatose. Even if I'm wrong, he will never achieve more than minimal mental function. Furthermore, since the respirator will not correct all of his life-threatening conditions, such as the severe anoxic brain damage, the intraventricular hemorrhage, and the kidney problem, I believe that treatment is futile, or at least virtually futile, and will merely prolong dying. If this were a voting committee, I would vote to turn off the respirator. Since we don't vote here, I would have no significant objection to this doctor's proposal.

"I think we may have already gone too far; if not, we will soon. This is another example of what I call the NICU two-step. One step down, a second sideways. We never have a final point in these infants, we just keep getting nibbled away to nothing. There's never one major crisis that we can't handle; there are always small crises that we can handle, and they keep adding up. Should we have resuscitated Castelli at birth when he showed evidence of severe hypoxia? Sure. It was easy to do, and he had a substantial chance for recovery. Should we have treated his seizures? Sure, that wasn't extraordinary and they weren't life threatening, even if they were evidence of a worse prognosis. Should we have treated his pneumothorax? Sure, we do that all the time. Untreated, it would be fatal; treated, his prognosis was unchanged. But it resulted in his intraventricular hemorrhage; we can't treat that, and his prognosis has gotten even worse. Now he has hydrocephalus. That has to be treated, since it's going to make his outlook worse and his care impossible. Treatment of the hydrocephalus brings in a whole new set of potential complications. Where do we stop? Where should we have stopped? It's all these little crises that end up as one big disaster."

"Mrs. Adams, I believe you had your hand up."

"It is not for you doctors to decide on the quality of life or on the right to life. I, and my organization, firmly believe that every human being has the right to life and that right is God given. It is not up to you to take it away by turning off the respirator. Nor is it up to the parents. That would be a very self-serving decision, wouldn't it? It sure would be nice to get rid of this problem—go back to their world travels and fancy restaurants and then maybe have a beautiful, perfect blond girl who would wear dresses from Saks. But that's too bad. God decided otherwise and put this baby here for His purposes, just as He put you physicians here to treat disease. Maybe this infant will enjoy his life, however long it may be. Perhaps this struggle will make the parents stronger and better people. Your job as physicians is not to judge lest you be judged, but to treat the infant as you treat so many infants in the nursery—with the best medicine and machines available and with your God-given wisdom."

"What is ethically right for Castelli, or any other infant, is the best quality of life possible—one that will bring the infant sufficient joy and happiness. Only if the infant can't achieve a sufficient level should we consider death a better alternative," began Scott Armstrong, the hospital's ethicist.

"I fully realize that these Baby Doe regulations prohibit our considering the quality of life, but that is patently ridiculous. Life is about quality. We allow adults to make decisions about the quality of their own lives. They can refuse treatment if they believe that quality is insufficient. They can even commit suicide if they don't like the quality of their lives. The only difference here is that Castelli is too young to assess the quality of his current and future life and is unable to articulate his thoughts. Everyone on this committee would agree that his current life is miserable. The quality of his future life doesn't smell like a rose either. Objectively, this quality of life is so poor that it is inhumane to continue life support."

"Scott," interjects Dr. Gross, "isn't that a very subjective assessment? I'm an opera buff. Life without the Met would have a much poorer quality, perhaps not even be worth living. I'll bet that few others on the committee would attach such importance to music.

"Music may be my major source of happiness. Life without music may be sufficiently poor that I could decide to end it. I can't make that assessment for you, but most of our colleagues seem to derive sufficient happiness from other sources that they consider their lives worth living, even without the Met."

"Sure it's difficult to assess what gives other people happiness or pleasure," says Armstrong. "Different people derive pleasure from varied things. It's difficult to determine the weight given to each. For some it might be just watching the sun rise that gives pleasure. Would that be sufficient pleasure to continue living? But we would all agree that for life to be worth living there must be some pleasure, joy, happiness and, however much there is, it must outweigh the pain."

"Scott, I agree with you. It doesn't look to me as if this Castelli baby has much happiness now," states Dr. Kendrick. "He's got all kinds of tubes and monitors, probably a headache from his hydrocephalus, and can't even derive happiness from being held like other babies while he's in an isolette. That's as poor a quality of life as I can conceive. That's just why I agree we should quit."

"You may be right, Ed," states one of the other committee members, "but that's a very shortsighted approach. If you had a heart attack and were in the ICU you might be just like Castelli. But when you recovered, you would probably come back to your old feisty self. So you can't look at quality of life only from the short term; you have to look at the future potential for happiness as well. I'll grant your argument about his current quality of life, and even the crises that may come up in the near future, but what about his potential to get better and grow up?"

"His future potential is grim. He has a high probability of severe retardation and severe cerebral palsy. He is likely to require operations to remove part of his bowel and also for his hydrocephalus. He has a reasonable likelihood of poor or nonexistent vision from retrolental fibroplasia. Is that a grim enough future for you?"

"You keep using the terms 'probability' and 'likelihood,' Ed. If we're making life-and-death decisions, don't we need certainty? Death is very final. We'd better be certain that we are right."

"There are very few certainties in medicine," responds Kendrick. "You know that. The overwhelming probability is that this infant is going to be a vegetable."

"Wait just a minute," interrupts Mrs. Adams. "Let's look at his happiness. Would he have any happiness if he was as you described? Could he experience any joy and pleasure? Is it possible or probable that he would at least look up at his mother's face and smile responsively? Could he show pleasure at being held or talked to? If he was able to do even these little things, who are we to say that they wouldn't be sufficient for him? Doesn't your utilitarian approach say that we should maximize even these little pleasures?"

"Who gives you the right to say that these minimal pleasures are sufficient?" asks George Lear, who represents the Council for the Disabled. "My daughter has a very full life in her wheelchair, but I don't think that merely smiling at society would be sufficient for her. Why do we always make the presumption that if we can't know decisively what a severely impaired individual would choose, that we always have to choose life? Maybe we're sentencing the individual who can't choose to 40 years of hell instead of going quickly to heaven. Isn't that equally possible?"

"The burden of proof always has to be on the side of those who would deny the right to life," rejoins Lucille Adams. "Otherwise, there would

135

always be the potential for abuse. We would get rid of all sorts of inconvenient people by claiming that they would be happier in heaven."

"You're pretty sure of your position, aren't you, Lucille? Wouldn't you at least admit the possibility that life could be hell and death a relief? Religion has preached and people have believed for centuries in 'the better life beyond.' " Lear sits back in his chair.

"This argument isn't getting us anywhere," states Kendrick. "Even if we grant that a smile is sufficient, what about its costs? Don't utilitarians have to count those? Look at the costs to the family. This baby will ruin their future lives. Look at the cost to society—the cost of what they call 'schooling' for these kids. The cost of physical therapy, stimulation, and all those things. Don't they outweigh the minimal pleasure for the baby?"

"Suppose this family wants the baby treated. Suppose that despite the prognosis the family wants to take him home. How would you deal with the social cost arguments then?" asks Lucille, smiling. "You wouldn't, would you? You'd just go on and treat. Well, let me tell you, if this family doesn't want the baby, I can find families who do. Families who would give him good care and derive much pleasure from doing so, whether or not he smiles."

"As chairman of this committee, it's time for me to bring the meeting to a close. Since this is an advisory committee, we don't have to vote. Let me sum up my impressions. We certainly have heard vigorous opinions from all sides. The argument that carried the most weight with me was Dr. Kendrick's statement that the key phrase in the regulations is 'a reasonable physician.' We would all agree that Dr. Kendrick is a reasonable physician; he clearly would turn off the respirator. I believe that I am also a reasonable physician and I believe, as I stated at the beginning, that treatment should be continued. You and the parents are going to have to decide which reasonable approach to take. In the past the courts have declined to overturn a decision made by parents who have chosen one of two reasonable options. Thank you all for your thoughtful and vigorous input."

* * *

You are a reasonable physician. What are you going to do? Whatever you are going to propose, you will have to defend your position on rounds tomorrow. If you want to stop treatment, you will have to convince Dr. Bernstein. If you want to continue treatment, you will have to face Dr. Kendrick. In either case, you will have to explain the pros and cons of your decision so that the students on rounds will learn. Outline your discussion for rounds tomorrow.

Chapter *13*

Amanda

"If it's a boy, let's name him Roger Farnsworth after both our fathers. If it's a girl, how about Amanda Lee? Amanda has always been my favorite girl's name. I hope it's a girl. I could teach her to cook and to sew. I can hardly wait. Can we get a piano? She should play the piano—'Amanda Roberts will now play the Rachmaninoff Piano Concerto in A Minor.' It's so exciting, I can't wait. Just three more weeks."

Saint Joseph's Memorial Hospital

Neurology Service Note   *Dr. S. Pert, Senior Resident*
Amanda Lee Roberts
Chief Complaint: Enlarging head
Birth Date: 10/23   Age: 4 days

Consult
  Requested because of full fontanelle and enlargement of the head.

History
  Full term; uneventful pregnancy. C-section for prolonged labor. First child. Father, age 31—lawyer. Mother, age 29—housewife. Family history negative. No problems during pregnancy, no fever, rash, vomiting. Delivery easy. Apgar 8/9. Doing well, feeding only fair.

Physical Examination
  Well-formed baby. Somewhat lethargic. Head circumference 39 centimeter (greater than 98 percentile). General exam okay. Heart good,

lungs clear. Abdomen normal. Fontanelle full. Eye movements okay, fundi normal, reflexes 2+ equal. Tone okay, moves all extremities.

Impression

Normal infant, possible hydrocephalus. Suggest CT or ultrasound scan before discharge.

Saul Pert, Senior Resident, Neurology

Dr. McDonald, Amanda's pediatrician, is one of the best-liked physicians at St. Joe's. A bear of a man, he is as gentle and jovial as he is large—a good doctor, who knows how to handle patients, parents, and problems. When you called him about your exam and recommendation, he was about to go hunting.

"Saul, my boy, do me a favor," he said. "Tell Mrs. Roberts that we want to get a scan and see if you can set it up for me. If the scan is okay, they can go home tomorrow. Tell Mrs. Roberts I'll see her in the morning."

Fortunately, there was an opening on the CT schedule that afternoon, and you make the arrangements. Just after 3 P.M. you receive a stat page to radiology. "Saul, get down here. You've got to see the scan on Roberts. You won't believe it."

The scan shows a big black space, and that is virtually all. Perhaps there is a small rim of brain up front, but the rest of the head is filled with fluid. The radiologist calls it hydranencephaly. How could a baby look so normal with so little brain? You decide you'd better read about hydranencephaly before you see the Roberts. McDonald wouldn't be back until tomorrow morning, and the Roberts aren't the type to wait for results until then.

You pull a text on pediatric neurology from your office shelf and read:

> Hydranencephaly is a rare condition in which the cortex of the brain either does not form or dissolves in utero. The infant with hydranencephaly, like the infant with anencephaly, has a normal brainstem and deep brain structures, so they are able to breath and survive, but the cortex, the locus of higher brain functions, is missing. The cause of hydranencephaly is unknown. For some it is believed that the cortex does not form and that this is the most extreme form of schizencephaly, but for most it is believed that the brain formed normally, but some event in the last trimester of pregancy, caused a major drop in blood supply to the fetal brain. The cortical tissue then died and was reabsorbed. This would explain the normal size

and shape of the head at birth. Hydrocephalus is common in these infants, and enlargement of the head is a common reason for studies which lead to the diagnosis. Despite the lack of cortical tissue, these infants may live for months or years, but have no capacity to make intellectual or motor progress.

You shut the book and think about what you will tell the Roberts. You decide that it's always best to tell the truth, but not necessarily the whole truth. You can play dumb and leave the really bad news for McDonald to deliver tomorrow.

"Mrs. Roberts, Mr. Roberts, it's a pleasure to meet you. I'm the senior resident in neurology. Dr. McDonald asked me to arrange the CT scan for Amanda and to tell you the results. He said he'd be back first thing in the morning. The scan shows some abnormalities, and I'm not completely sure what they mean. I'll have to go over them with Dr. McDonald, and he can talk with you tomorrow morning."

"Are they bad? It isn't anything serious, is it? We're supposed to go home tomorrow."

"I've told you about all I know, Mrs. Roberts. We'll just have to wait until the morning."

Dr. McDonald stops at the nursery about 8 A.M., reads your note in Amanda's chart, and pages you. "Meet me in radiology and let's go over the scan together," he says.

"Damnation, will you look at that!" says McDonald when you put the scans on the viewing board. "There's nothing in that head but water. I don't think I've seen anything like that since I was a resident. You know, that baby looks so normal; her exam is perfect. I thought she might have a bit of hydrocephalus. I guess I'd better get Ron in here; he's seen about all the neurosurgical problems that exist. He'll know what to do and what to tell the family.

Dr. Culver takes one look and says, "Throw it back and try again. This child has no future. She's like an anencephalic infant except she doesn't look so bad. There's nothing that can be done."

"What happens to these kids?" asks McDonald.

"Some die soon, but some live for months. They often develop hydrocephalus, and their heads get larger and larger. If you shunt them they live longer; if you don't they become nursing care problems. Heads you lose, tails you lose."

"Thanks for coming in, Ron, and thanks for the information."

"Robin, Jack, good morning," began Dr. McDonald. "I've been down looking at Amanda's scan from yesterday and I've gone over it with the neurosurgeon. I'm afraid that we've got a problem. The scan shows bad damage to her brain, very bad damage. Something happened before she was born. It was nothing you did or didn't do. We don't know the cause, but this is one of the few situations where we can say with confidence that an infant will be severely retarded. There's nothing we can do except hope and pray. Let me explain in a bit more detail."

Robin is weeping in Jack's arms. "She's so beautiful. I can't believe it. What are we going to do, Jack? Can we take her home? The nursery is all ready for her. My mother's coming in today to help. Will she be able to walk, Dr. McDonald? Will she talk?"

"I'm afraid that both of those things are unlikely, my dear. Amanda may not even be able to see. Her eyes are fine, but the seeing part of the brain is badly damaged. Yes, you can take her home. For now she's just like any other newborn. The problem is that she will stay that way. Many of these infants don't survive too long, and that may be a blessing. Some develop hydrocephalus—water on the brain. We can worry about that later.

"Why don't you get dressed and take her home? I'll come by your house tomorrow and we can talk some more."

Three weeks later, at the first official well-baby check, the head is growing far too rapidly. Forty-six centimeters, the size it should be at 9 months of age. There is little doubt about the hydrocephalus. Other than that, things have gone rather well. Dr. McDonald has talked with the Roberts a number of times. They seem to be coping and adjusting better than many families. They obviously love Amanda and are giving her excellent care.

Dr. McDonald arranges to meet you and Dr. Culver after ward rounds; the pediatric residents join you.

"Ron, remember Amanda Roberts, the baby with hydranencephaly?" asks Dr. McDonald. "I saw her yesterday and her head is growing off the chart. It's 46 centimeters already. Shouldn't we put in a shunt to control the hydrocephalus and the size of her head?"

"Well, Joe," says Dr. Culver, "you'll be damned if you do and damned if you don't. If you do you can keep the head a manageable size. But, as you know, the shunts get blocked up or infected, and you'll have to decide about fixing it time after time. And the shunt won't make her better; it will just make her live longer. If you don't shunt her she'll live shorter, but even that may be a long time."

"Dr. Culver," one of the residents asks, "does the intracranial pressure cause her pain? Will she suffer if we don't put in a shunt?"

"That's hard to say, son," he responds. "She hasn't got many ways of showing pain, but she hasn't got much brain to feel pain either. She's just a human form, a shell, not a person. It's a shame, she is a pretty baby."

"Thanks for your time, Ron," says Dr. McDonald. "I guess I'll talk it over with her folks and decide what to do. If they want the operation I'll give you a call."

The Philosophical Society

The third Thursday night of each month the Winona County Philosophical Society meets in the county library. Discussions are free floating, since there is no fixed agenda. You were a philosophy major in college, and membership in the Society offers a welcome relief from the medical chores of your residency.

When you arrived about 8 P.M., only Professor Bagley from State was there. Others would doubtless arrive shortly.

"How's the world of medicine, young man?" asks Professor Bagley. "Keeping you busy, or do you still have time to exercise your mind?" Bagley's view of doctors is not one of admiration.

"Let me ask you a question, Professor," you begin. "We were discussing a patient the other day, and during the discussion I wondered if she was a person. Did she qualify as a human being? I've been thinking about it since and trying to define personhood, the quality of humanness."

"That's a pretty tough problem for a doctor to think about," says Bagley. "Seriously, that is a topic we philosophers have been working on. Aristotle defined man as the rational animal. Descartes claimed that man is a thinking thing. While 'thinking' or 'rational' are hard terms to define, they appear to be essential ingredients of what makes us people."

"Wait a minute, professor," you interrupt. "Thinking can't be what makes a person. What about the chimps who can use symbols and computers to communicate? Dolphins seem to reason. Even my dog is smart and at times seems quite rational. No one is going to say that any of these animals are human."

"Let me clarify," replies Bagley. "Humans, the human race, is defined by biologic and genetic characteristics in the same sense that we define codfish or sparrows or any other species. Personhood is a moral rather than a biological category, and most people hold that thinking and rationality are essential to it.

"Personhood has an interesting history. In the U.S. Constitution slaves were counted as three fifths of a person. Even in the late nineteenth century, American Indians were not counted or treated as persons at all. Women were persons but did not have the rights of male persons, and prisoners had even fewer rights. But the argument recently surfaced over fetuses and comatose adults."

"Professor, are you saying that humanness and personhood are not the same thing? That humanness is genetic, while personhood is acquired or bestowed?"

"Yes, that's exactly what I'm saying. The importance of bestowing personhood is that with personhood we bestow rights, different rights to different persons, to be sure, but some rights."

"Who bestows these rights? For that matter, who bestows personhood?"

"Well, philosophers disagree about that. Some have felt that personhood comes with the genetic traits, some have felt that it comes from God. Others feel that it's bestowed by those who have it, those who are already members of the club.

"Recently there have been arguments about the adult in coma. At what point does this comatose human being lose personhood and become just a warm body? This is an important question because at some point the individual may lose the rights to our services and we may lose our obligation to continue them."

"Bagley, are you discussing personhood again? Have you gotten to the part about newborn and potential persons yet?"

"It's about time you got here, Martha," says Bagley. "Doctor, this is Martha Appelby, the minister at the First Unitarian Church. Martha, this young man is raising some important questions."

"Let me tell you about the infant who brought this whole issue up," you say. "She's now about 4 weeks old and, to all appearances, a very pretty little girl, except her head is a bit large. Other than that you wouldn't know anything was wrong. But it turns out she has no brain, at least no cortex. We can establish, without question, that she cannot see, cannot hear (or at least will never be able to understand sounds) and, without a cortex, will never think. Thus, she has no awareness of her environment and no potential to develop even minimal human relationships. The question is, is she a person?"

"Well, that gets us into all those arguments about newborns and potential persons," says Martha. "Right now she's not much different than any other newborn, is she? Newborns are considered persons even when they don't have any demonstrable capacity for thinking, rationality, or relating to others. Since they have the potential to develop these capacities, we give them a certificate of personhood at birth. Maybe we shouldn't. Maybe we should wait a period of time until the infant has realized some potential.

"My quandary," you respond, "is what to do for this infant. She has hydrocephalus and the question is whether to put in a shunt to prolong her life and make it easier to take care of her while she exists. The other choice would be not to do the operation, which will allow her to die sooner but will make it more difficult to take care of her in the meantime."

"Would it make a difference if you considered her a person?" asks Martha.

"No, I guess not," you reply. "I have to do what's best for her and her family, when we decide what that is."

"How about if you considered her a nonperson?" asks Professor Bagley.

"Well, I've never thought of another human as a nonperson. I suppose if I were a veterinarian and someone brought in a puppy, I'd still want to do what was best for the dog. Sometimes, of course, I would put a puppy out of its misery or even dispose of. . . ."

At this point your beeper sounds, insistently signaling a stat page to the emergency room. You rush out past several members of the Society who are about to enjoy the discussion you started.

*   *   *

Think about the personhood arguments presented. Do they help you in your thinking about Amanda and her management? Would they have been helpful in your decisions about the termination of care of Edgar Jones (Chapter 7)? When dealing with infants with severe brain damage but with less certain outcome, would personhood arguments be more or less helpful? How do you reconcile arguments about personhood with arguments about rights and duties to respect?

What would you do if it was your job to advise the parents? Is it better to keep Amanda's head close to normal size so that she appears more normal and nursing care will be made easier? Is it better to do nothing and hope she dies quickly, even though that may make her care more difficult in the intervening weeks or months? Does Amanda have any right to one approach or the other? What is in her best interest? What effect do the arguments about personhood have on your decision?

Chapter 14

Ethical Theory
and Medical Ethics

Defining "Morals" and "Ethics"

In both popular and professional language, the terms *moral* and *ethical* are used in several senses. Public officials are sometimes guilty of un-ethical behavior, while people who violate a law dealing with sexual ac-tivity are arrested on morals charges. College courses on ethics are often taught by moral philosophers. Although the term *moral* is sometimes used as a word of praise, as in "she is a very moral person," on other occa-sions it has a much wider meaning.

In this and the following chapter we use the word *moral* to refer to the actions or activities for which a certain kind of praise or blame is awarded. Morally good actions are marked, for example, by courage, wisdom, balance, or fairness, while morally bad or immoral actions are characterized by opposite qualities. We use *morality* to refer to the col-lection of an individual's or a society's moral actions.

We praise people for many things, such as their intelligence or atheletic ability. Some people excel in sports or in school primarily on native ability. While we admire or even envy such people, we have a different kind of admiration for people who bring certain personal attributes to whatever they do. As the cliché says, "It matters not whether you win or lose, it's how you play the game."

The outer box of Figure 14-1 diagrams all human activity. Moral ac-tivity falls inside the circle; activity or behavior outside the moral circle is amoral or morally neutral, neither good nor bad. We do innumerable amoral things all the time, such as breathe, chew gum, and sleep.

OUTLINE OF ALL HUMAN ACTIVITY

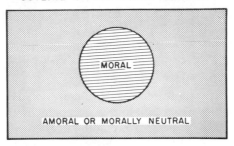

Figure 14-1.

The borders of morally significant activity are, however, notoriously hard to define. They are themselves matters of substantial controversy. Are smoking, taxpaying, or gambling morally neutral and indifferent, or are they part of the kind of person one is? There is controversy about where these examples would fit into our picture; some people claim that smoking, for example, is just an amoral habit, while others say that since it is known to be harmful to one's health, the decision to smoke is part of one's moral makeup.

Moral activity is not exotic; it is something we do every day. Discussion or argument about morality is also very ordinary. We evaluate the actions of others, and we think critically about ourselves. We are concerned about how people evaluate us and even more about how we really are. As we define it, *ethics* is the discussion about and theory of morality. Whenever we discuss morals, we appeal either implicitly or explicitly to theories justifying our judgments. Ethics, as Figure 14-2 shows, is like a grid that fits over our moral activity.

OUTLINE OF ALL HUMAN ACTIVITY

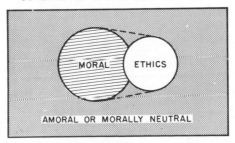

Figure 14-2.

145

Defining ethics and morality as we do makes some matters a little clearer. For example, failing a course in ethics need not be a moral disgrace. In fact, people may fail for admirable reasons, such as missing classes and assignments to care for a sick parent. Furthermore, taking a course in ethics may help someone see the issues of morality a little more clearly than they otherwise might have. There is no guarantee, naturally, that a course will produce better people, nor is a medical school requirement in medical ethics likely to improve dramatically the morality of the physicians who take the course. Defining the terms this way also accounts for the fact that some philosophers who know a lot about ethical theory are not admirable people and that some morally upstanding people know very little or nothing about ethical theory.

The case studies in this book, so far as possible, make you a participant in moral decision making. They also help you to realize that discussing these matters makes you an ethical theorist whether or not you relish that role. The theories we are about to discuss are not merely abstract possibilities or bright ideas from far away and long ago. They are ways in which people in the late twentieth century actually discuss with each other what should be done and also ways in which we think about ourselves and how we act.

Throughout the cases we have involved you in the process of making moral decisions. The following discussion of ethical theory is designed to help you think about what you are doing. We hope and expect that thinking about the reasons for making decisions, and understanding how others might think about them, will help in making better decisions. Ethics, as we are concerned with it, is not a theory for outsiders to moral decision making. Since morality is not a spectator sport, ethics, as we deal with it, is a theory of morality for participants.

Ethics, therefore, is not as separate from morality as what we said previously might first suggest. What people do is strongly influenced by what they think, and how they think is much influenced by what they do. All of us are involved both in morality and in ethics. We have all been speaking ethics for a long time; reviewing ethical theory should help us to speak better.

Public and Private Morality

Just as distinguishing between ethics and morality can clarify our discussion, distinguishing *public* from *private* morality can save a great deal of confusion (see Fig. 14-3).

The problems of medical ethics are especially vexing because they live on the border between public and private morality. Unlike issues of

OUTLINE OF ALL HUMAN ACTIVITY

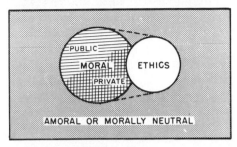

Figure 14-3.

racism or capital punishment, which are clearly public, and attitudes of personal respect or control of one's temper, which are clearly private, the problems of medical ethics thrive in the overlap between these two areas of morality. Patients often claim control over their medical care on the grounds that their decisions are private, yet the very privacy of those decisions is protected by the public practices of the medical profession and by government regulation. The conflict between public and private morality is a key ingredient in many of the cases presented here.

The tension between public and private morality exists between two sides of morality, not between the moral and the amoral. Abortion is a good example of an issue that lives on this border. One may argue against abortion both as a private choice and as public policy, or one may argue that abortion has positive value as a private choice and should be tolerated or even encouraged as public policy. One may also take a mixed position, arguing against abortion as a private choice, but in favor of toleration as public policy or even in favor of funding it for the poor as a matter of justice. Both the public and private sides of these positions are moral stances that invite ethical scrutiny.

One needs, therefore, to develop an ethical theory that provides for a reasonable relationship between public and private concerns. Therefore, as we discuss ethical theories in the following sections, we will describe how they deal with the tensions between public and private morality. The ability of an ethical theory to deal with this issue is one measure of its success.

Distinguishing Good from Bad Morality

The most important measure of the success of an ethical theory, however, is its ability to distinguish morally good from morally bad actions

OUTLINE OF ALL HUMAN ACTIVITY

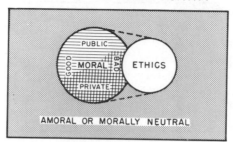

Figure 14-4.

(Fig. 14-4). As one would expect, drawing this distinction is a matter of intense philosophical argument.

Since the early part of the nineteenth century, ethics has been dominated by two approaches to distinguishing good from bad. Utilitarianism, developed by Jeremy Bentham and John Stuart Mill, judges the morality of actions by the happiness they generate. Theories of rights and duties (often called *deontological* theories), developed under the inspiration of Immanuel Kant, hold that adherence to duty is the primary measure of moral goodness. Both are "single-key" theories because they argue that there is one fundamental test of the moral rightness of any course of action. Both theories work to apply their distinctive rule to what should be done in given situations. They do not start with judgments about good character and the good life as many ancient and medieval philosophers did, nor do they start with the social and economic system as Karl Marx did. These single-key theories focus on the actions of individuals. They try to answer the question "What should I do?" For that reason we call them *what theories*. The next three sections will deal with the most prominent of these theories.

Utilitarianism

Utilitarianism was developed by a group of late eighteenth- and nineteenth-century British philosophers. In the classic phrase of John Stuart Mill, a nineteenth-century philosopher and social reformer, a utilitarian considers those acts to be right that "produce the greatest happiness for the greatest number." Although there are many variations on this theme, utilitarian theories have certain common characteristics.

First, they are *consequentialist*. The rightness of an action is measured by the value of its consequences, what happens as a result of the action.

148

Since all actions have both good and bad consequences, it is more precise to say that utilitarianism is a theory of *proportionality,* meaning that the best action has the highest proportion of good to bad consequences. *Cost/benefit* analysis and other tools of contemporary economics and management have evolved from utilitarian thinking. Many medical decisions also use cost/benefit analysis. In the medical situation, the costs are not simply monetary but include psychological, social, and physical effects.

Second, utilitarian theories define good actions as those that produce a good that the theory specifies. Determining the proportion between good and bad consequences requires some notion of what good consequences are. Utilitarian theorists all develop such a concept, whether it be Jeremy Bentham's narrow concept of pleasure, happiness (which the Greeks called *eudaimonia*), or more contemporary views about quality of life. Good actions, in the utilitarian view, are those that proportionally produce more good than any alternative.

Utilitarianism has the advantage of somehow feeling right. Pain and unhappiness are surely not good things and should be minimized, while pleasure, happiness, love, joy, and fulfillment are good things. Most people feel that good actions should produce happiness, not misery.

Moreover, utilitarianism promises to decide moral issues rationally. It is satisfying to add up the good consequences of an action on one side and the bad on another to arrive at a rational decision. Much modern decision theory and analysis of medical therapy, not to mention common sense, are based on such an approach. Utilitarianism tries to develop a clear bottom line for good decisions.

Characters in several of our cases advocate utilitarian decision making. Often, as with Christie or the Castelli baby, the philosopher member of the ethics committee advocates a utilitarian approach. The utilitarian weighs the likelihood of good or bad outcomes for the patient, the family, society, and others to arrive at the best decision for all concerned.

Carrying out the utilitarian program, however, turns out to be a complicated business. As medical situations shift and change, both costs and benefits are hard to predict. Utilitarians deal with such uncertainty by adding a factor to their calculations. This factor is called *risk, probability,* or *chance.* Utilitarians try to compare the risk of high costs to the risk of low benefits. For example, the utilitarian compares the risk of costly medical care and bad outcome to the chance of moderately expensive medical care and good outcome, the risks of physical and psychosocial costs to patient and family to the pleasures and benefits of each. A probability factor must be assigned to each of the more common complications of treatment. A negative or positive value can thus be assigned to each proposed course of action.

149

When we first encounter utilitarianism, the kind of thinking it requires seems straightforward and commonsensical. It seems to be the same kind of thinking we might use to decide which of three or four apartments to rent or which model car to buy. As we try to analyze cases using utilitarian calculations, however, the work becomes increasingly difficult, more like weighing risks involved in various methods of nuclear deterrence than a common practical decision. How does one weigh the risks and benefits of ICBMs, cruise missiles, strategic bombers, multiple warheads, and the strategic defense initiative? Utilitarianism is not as easy to apply as might at first appear.

Since utilitarianism focuses on results or consequences, such theories are the target of the traditional challenge, "Does the end justify the means?" The utilitarian argues that if the result of two different actions is the same, the actions and their morality are the same. From a utilitarian perspective, the ends arrived at are precisely what justify whatever means are used. If a utilitarian concludes that it is best for a patient to die, any distinctions among the means, for example, between *killing* and *letting die,* become unimportant. In discussions of euthanasia the utilitarian argues that the difference between killing a patient and letting the patient die is mainly the terrible costs in pain and suffering for both patient and family that letting die often involves.

Finally, the utilitarian does not limit the calculation of costs and benefits to those of the patient. While the principal costs and benefits may be the patient's, there are always others to be considered: family, other caretakers, the medical care system, and society as a whole. If utilitarianism insists that we act for the benefit of the greatest number, we must include all, even perhaps future generations, as factors in our calculations.

Taking the social context into account is both the greatest strength and the greatest weakness of utilitarianism. The theory recognizes that the public and the private spheres are closely connected and that individual decisions have wide-ranging social consequences. There was a day when health care decisions were strictly between physician and patient, but such simplicity no longer applies. Many areas of medicine are not as private as they used to be. Utilitarians argue that good decisions must take account of the consequences for families, the medical care system, employers, insurance companies, the government—in short, the whole society. The willingness of utilitarianism to take account of these factors, however, gives rise to one of the classic objections to the theory.

Utilitarianism sometimes seems to demand that we sacrifice some good, perhaps even the life, of an individual because that person's life is so "expensive" to other people. If a person's life is some, but only a small, benefit to himself and a great burden to others, the greatest happiness of the greatest number will be secured by sacrificing the individual. If terrorists, for example, demand that a government official be killed or they will use a nuclear bomb to destroy a major city, the utilitarian seems compelled to sacrifice one to save many. If Christie or the Castelli baby will lead only a marginal life while making their parents' lives miserable and placing a great burden on society then, by utilitarian theory, it is best to see that they do not survive.

Some utilitarians have tried to deal with such violations of customary morality by developing a variation called *rule utilitarianism.* (Whether rule utilitarianism is a genuinely distinct theory or just a long-range version of the original, or *act utilitarian,* theory is a controversial question among philosophers.) Rule utilitarians argue that we should not judge individual actions but rather social rules, institutions, or practices. There are immediate benefits of giving in to terrorists, but the costs of the social practice of appeasement might easily outweigh them. The reverse may be said of the care of individuals. While Christie's care, viewed as a series of isolated acts, might be too expensive, the practice of providing costly care for the handicapped might provide an overall benefit to society.

Rule utilitarianism thus takes account of other moral traditions, notably that of individual rights. It can argue that the notion of rights that is central to many ethical arguments is only a quick way of expressing good social practices. The right to free speech, for example, is well justified by its results in opening communication in society and enhancing individual satisfaction. The utilitarian, however, argues that rights are not absolutes but are limited in situations in which honoring them would produce harmful consequences. The standard example is that the right of free speech does not protect someone who falsely cries "Fire!" in a crowded theater. Individual rights, the utilitarian claims, are social practices that are beneficial in the long run.

Several of our cases turn on a conflict between a benefit for the individual or society and some standard notion of rights or duties that seems to prohibit obtaining the benefit, or at least obtaining it in a certain way. In thinking about euthanasia in the case of Edgar Jones, for example, the utilitarian compares the poor quality of Edgar's life with the great costs of keeping him alive. Utilitarians interpret the discussion of the rights of Edgar or his wife to make a decision, or about the duties of physicians as merely a way of arguing about the consequences of active euthanasia. They argue that their way of thinking about the issue, their ethical theory, is clearer and keeps our attention where it should be, on the good and bad consequences of each proposed course of action.

No matter with which version of utilitarianism one works, however, the question remains whether it can handle the objection that it sacrifices individuals and their integrity to some wider good. The utilitarian takes individual rights to be no more than instruments of social benefit and individual integrity merely a means of producing good. For unmixed utilitarians there is finally no question but that individuals, whether themselves or others, should be sacrificed for the good of the whole. Recognizing this objection, most current forms of utilitarianism introduce some additional principles to dilute the impact of the theory on individuals.

Classical utilitarians, however, can deal with this objection by claiming that some of our moral intuitions are faulty and should be reconstituted in a utilitarian fashion. After all, the function of an ethical theory is to organize and systematize our morality. All of our present moral beliefs should not come through the process unchanged. Utilitarians can also point out that their theory at least accords with one of our basic intuitions about morality: that it should lead to human happiness. Rights and duties, they may claim, are not moral absolutes but make sense only when placed in the service of happiness.

While agreeing with the utilitarian that human well-being and fulfillment are crucial to morality, we part from the claim that the concept of human happiness can be developed sufficiently to provide a moral "bottom line" or single standard against which the goodness of actions can be measured. The notion of good or happiness is too rich and ambiguous to provide such a standard. Some people cling to lives that very few would consider worth living, while others who seem to live full and satisfying lives reject them with self-destructive behavior. The term "quality of life" has a nice ring, but it becomes entirely too vague when people try to apply it to actual situations. It does not seem possible to develop a sufficiently defined and acceptable notion of good or benefit to allow someone to evaluate consequences as utilitarianism demands. As Mr. McBundy points out to the ethics committee considering Christie's case, different alternatives for Christie's care can be weighed differently by different people.

Even if there were a precise way to define happiness, working with utilitarian calculations would be a nightmare. Because every action has endless consequences, calculating the costs and benefits of alternative possibilities becomes a herculean task. Introducing risk further complicates the calculations. Several cases in this book show the difficulty of predicting outcome, especially when one tries to take account of improvements that might be brought about by new therapies. When, for example, the statistics for survival with untreated spina bifida are so poorly established and the lives or deaths of the treated and the untreated are so unpredictably diverse, how does the utilitarian calculate whether or not to treat Christie?

Finally, the utilitarian claim that happiness or fulfillment is the ultimate value against which any other value can be measured fails to give adequate importance to staples of our moral thinking such as rights and personal integrity. As the existentialists and others have observed, freedom and its accompanying responsibility do not always make people happy, but they are still part of our human dignity. Utilitarianism is too ready to see individuals, their rights, and their integrity merely as means to happiness without an inherent value of their own.

To draw some examples from the cases in this book, knowledge of one's family history of Huntington's disease in the "Smyth Saga" is not, for the utilitarian, a matter of right but only a function of what makes people happy. Because we do not always know what will make us happy, however, others must make a judgment about what we should know based on their ideas of how we will feel. Since the utilitarian evaluates actions on the results they bring, the impact of a decision on the person who decides has no special place among the many effects of any action. In "Tom Revisited," the utilitarian views Rosa's involvement in making decisions about her son only as a function of her feeling about what is happening to Tom. Because it concentrates on the results of decisions, the effect of decisions on the people who make them is only one of innumerable effects of an action. Actions and their consequences are what matter, not actors and their integrity.

These objections to utilitarianism are neither original nor, as we have stated them, fatal to the theory. Their force, however, is to make the theory less obvious. Also, the objections are raised to utilitarianism as an ethical theory, that is, to a way of thinking about morality. We are not criticizing it for giving the wrong results but, at least taken by itself, for being an inadequate way to think about moral issues.

Please do not be satisfied, moreover, with our introduction to these important arguments. There is a guide to further reading at the end of this chapter so that you can explore the ideas of utilitarians and their critics in their own terms. As you develop your own ethical position, we hope you work as closely as possible with the primary advocates of the major philosophical positions.

As we move beyond utilitarian theory, however, it will be well to take along the utilitarian's concern for human happiness and well-being. Some of the theories we are about to examine are so concerned with other aspects of morality that they neglect this essential element. We agree with the utilitarians that happiness and fulfillment must be part of our moral system; we only reject the consequentialist way utilitarians incorporate these realities in their theory.

The objections to utilitarianism naturally turn us to an ethics of duty.

Typical theories of duty pay a great deal of attention to the integrity and importance of the individual and, since they do not rest their moral evaluation on consequences, they do not get snarled in the objectionable calculations of utilitarianism.

The Theory of Duties

Contemporary theories of duty take their inspiration from the work of Immanuel Kant, a philosopher of the late eighteenth century. Like utilitarianism, Kant's theory proposes a single rule for judging the rightness or wrongness of an action, but Kant proposes a different rule of good action that he applies to a different aspect of moral activity.

One of the principal objections to utilitarianism turns on the difficulties of calculating the consequences of our decisions. As our cases make clear, no one has full control of the outcome, even with good medical practice. Many of the consequences of our action depend on chance, luck, or other factors outside our control. Because we only praise or blame people in a moral way for what they deliberately do, Kant argues that moral evaluation has to apply to something under our control. He therefore proposes that moral evaluation apply directly to the decision, to the decision-making act of the will, and not to consequences. As he puts it, "Nothing in the world—indeed nothing even beyond the world—can possibly be conceived which could be called good without qualification except a good will." Instead of looking at the consequences of actions, Kant focuses moral evaluation on the choice itself.

Kant calls the rule for judging good rules of action the *categorical imperative.* Although he phrased it in several ways, the clearest expression of the categorical imperative for our purposes is, "Act so that you treat humanity, both in your own person and in that of another, always as an end and never merely as a means." Contemporary philosophers often refer to this as the *respect principle,* the principle that demands human respect for other people and for ourselves. The respect that health care professionals owe their patients is a special case of the respect that every person owes every other.

Informed consent is a good example of the application of the respect principle. We have a duty to treat patients only with their consent because we have a moral obligation to respect their choices and free decisions. Obtaining consent treats patients as human beings, as people who exert control over their own lives, and not merely as objects or means to some purposes of ours. People have what Kant calls moral autonomy, the ability to make rules for themselves. In contrast with act utilitarianism, the Kantian does not think it critically important whether people are happier for being told of the side effects of their drugs or their risk of being victims of genetically transmitted disease. The theory of moral duty holds that people should be told such things as part of the respect that doctors and nurses owe their patients.

Kant argues that the respect principle is morally valid because it can be universally or categorically applied. If you do not want to be treated without your consent, lied to about your medical care, or treated as a child or an incompetent, you should not treat others that way. As the golden rule has it, treat others as you would be treated. Kant argues that it makes no sense to want to be treated in a paternalistic, condescending, or not-fully-human way, that it is virtually self-contradictory to say "lie to me." Furthermore, there is no justification for treating people in similar circumstances differently from one another. The Kantian perspective in medical ethics, therefore, has strongly criticized paternalism or benevolent lying while emphasizing truth telling, autonomy, and informed consent.

Kant's moral theory is *deontological* (derived from the Greek word for what one must do) because it uses the categorical imperative to develop a list of moral duties. The most general duties are binding on all human beings at all times.

Duties may be divided into *positive duties* and *negative duties*. Treating people with respect, for example, means at least that we should not lie to them. Not lying or not killing, therefore, are universal negative duties. In the tradition of the Hippocratic oath, the most important duty of the physician is "First, do no harm." The negative duty, expressed in the Biblical command as "Thou shalt not kill," is more fundamental and absolute than the obligation to give aid.

Positive duties, on the other hand, commit us to acting in certain ways. Positive obligations may be generated by explicit commitments, promises, or contracts or generated implicitly by social roles or customs. In an ethics of duty, physicians have a strong positive duty to patients they have accepted into their practices that is much stronger than to sick people in general. Nurses have similarly strong obligations to patients in a hospital for which they work. Hospitals also have special obligations to their patients and the local communities they serve.

Two examples illustrate the difference between positive and negative duties: the distinction between truth telling and lying and that between killing and letting die. Theories of moral duty hold that there is a very strong duty not to lie, but the positive duty to tell the truth is not as strong. In medical situations the duty to tell the truth is relative to many things, including the patient's level of understanding, physical and emotional condition, and desire to know. Cancer patients who ask pointed questions, for example, should be told the truth. Although there is a strong duty not to lie, the duty to tell the truth to those who do not seek it out, or who try to avoid it, is much weaker.

The distinction between positive and negative duties is also significant for its close connection to the distinction between killing and letting die, between active and passive euthanasia. Negative duties, since they are universally binding, have priority over positive ones. While not all theories of moral duty prohibit killing in every circumstance, they do recognize a substantial difference between killing and leveling off or reducing the level of medical care even while anticipating the patient's death. The positive obligation to provide medical care is relative to the technology available, the patient's condition and wishes, and the patient's relation to family and society. Although the duty to provide a certain level of medical care may depend on the circumstances, the duty not to kill is negative, definite, and much stronger. The outer limits of the duty to treat is not as strictly defined a moral requirement as the duty not to kill or harm.

Of course, theories of moral duty do not find every instance of letting die to be morally acceptable. The fact that not treating is not doing something, an *omission* rather than a *commission,* is irrelevant when there is a clear and positive duty to act. The case of Edgar Jones shows how problems arise as we move along the sliding scale of moral duty. If our duty to support and care for patients is a matter of degree, where is the line drawn in a case like Edgar's? How strong is the duty to put him on the respirator, to continue him on it, to provide nutrition and hydration? Different versions of moral duty theory offer various answers to such questions. Some argue that we should do everything medically possible because only maximum treatment is morally acceptable. Most theories, however, would accept something less than maximum intervention. Some would limit the duty to care by the duty to honor the patient's wishes or those of the family, while others would limit these duties by distinguishing between ordinary and extraordinary care. *Ordinary* care, in this view, is the level of care demanded by the duty to respect another human being. *Extraordinary* care is in some way optional for the patient or is beyond that which we are strictly obliged to provide.

Such distinctions separate theories of duty from utilitarianism. The moral evaluation of an action, the utilitarian argues, depends only on the balance of good to bad consequences. Whether a patient dies by commission or omission, after receiving ordinary or extraordinary care, or by active or passive euthanasia is simply not important. Because it focuses on consequences, utilitarianism argues that these distinctions only confuse our moral thought.

Codes of professional morality list the positive duties of health care providers. The American Nurses Association's Code for Nurses and the American Medical Association's Principles of Medical Ethics are two examples. Both begin by requiring practitioners to respect the human dignity of their patients (physicians) or clients (nurses). They then spell out what respect entails. Each of the codes requires that the patients' confidentiality be honored and that practitioners act to insure the integrity of health care by taking action in cases of incompetent or unethical practice.

The standard codes of professional morality and our conventional ideas of duty are, however, only indirectly related to the fundamental duty of human respect. When one gets down to cases, matters become difficult. First, the obligations listed in the codes of nursing or medical practice sometimes conflict. The duty to respect a client's confidences, for example, can conflict with the duty to take action against incompetent or unethical practice.

Moreover, our obligations are not usually precisely defined. No one is opposed to respecting human dignity as long as what that means is left unspecified. When the question of active euthanasia is argued, as in the case of Edgar Jones, some people hold that euthanasia respects the dignity of the patient because it respects the patient's wishes, while others argue that it destroys the dignity of health care professionals and undermines each person's duty to respect his or her own life.

An ethics of moral duty has several important strengths. First, grounding the respect principle with a golden rule argument is a very effective strategy. Second, the main duties of physicians and nurses, which are derived from the basic principle, are consonant with our fundamental moral intuitions, at least in their abstract expression. The problem with the theory of moral duties arises in the course of developing concrete moral guidance from the basic principle. In the abstract the theory has much to be said for it, but getting it to work for individual decisions raises some serious problems.

Before we can isolate the elements of a duty theory of morality that we want to retain, however, it is useful to sketch out a related theory—the theory of moral rights.

Moral Rights

The theory of duties and the theory of moral rights are usually thought of as the two sides of the same coin. If one has a right to something, someone else has the duty to deliver it, and any duties one might have generate corresponding rights in other people. If one accepts a patient into one's practice, the patient has a right to one's competent medical care. Likewise, the rights of patients generate duties. If patients have the right to know what is in their medical records, physicians or nurses in possession of the records have a duty to disclose the information.

While rights and duties are correlative, there is a great philosophical controversy about which one is primary. Some philosophers hold that rights generate duties; others insist that it goes the other way around. Generally, philosophers who begin from a social or political perspective tend to make rights primary, while those who start from the perspective of individual decisions tend to take duties as fundamental.

As shown in the previous section, starting from duties has the philosophical advantage of resting on a strong argument. Beginning with rights, on the other hand, provides a position with great rhetorical power. As one contemporary philosopher has phrased it, rights are "trump cards" that, when played, settle the issue in favor of the one playing them. People love having rights, and the more of them the better. No one can have too many rights. The same can hardly be said of duties; even one duty is sometimes too many. The founding documents of the United States are couched in terms of rights, dependent as they are on the thinking of natural rights theorists of the eighteenth century such as John Locke and Jean-Jacques Rousseau. In the words of the U.S. Declaration of Independence, "We hold these truths to be self-evident, that all men are created equal; that they are endowed by their Creator with certain inalienable rights; that among these are life, liberty, and the pursuit of happiness." This single sentence contains all the important elements of a theory of rights, and each element shows both the advantages and disadvantages of such a theory.

The first element of any theory of rights is the *scope* of the theory; who has the rights? The Declaration speaks of "all men," which in its historical context meant something close to "white, male property owners." In the U.S. Constitution, each slave was counted as three-fifths a person in determining the population of the states. The document assumes that women would not vote; it does not challenge the laws in various states limiting the right to vote to property owners or imposing a tax on voting. All these measures substantially restricted the scope of constitutional rights until well into this century.

In contemporary terms, the conflict over abortion and some cases of euthanasia is a conflict over the scope of rights. In *Roe* v. *Wade,* the U.S. Supreme Court held that since the issue was so variously debated by philosophers and theologians, no one can be sure that fetuses incapable of surviving outside the womb are really persons. Since only persons have constitutional rights, fetuses could not be said to have such rights during the first two trimesters of their mothers' pregnancy. The Supreme Court went on to rule that because fetuses fell outside the scope of full human rights, abortion during the first two trimesters was a private right of women that could not be prohibited by state or federal law.

The second element of a theory of rights is the *source* or origin of the rights. The framers of the U.S. Constitution held that God gave people rights. The theological argument is widely criticized today by both believers and nonbelievers. Many Christians point out that biblical ethics says more about duties or God's love than it does about rights. Religious people from other traditions observe that the theory of rights is not part of their heritage, while nonbelievers observe that attempting to ground rights on a religious basis compromises the theory by threatening it with sectarian strife.

Contemporary defenses of rights either omit the question of origins, which weakens them philosophically, or defend rights as derived from some version of the respect principle. Deriving rights from the respect principle, however, subordinates rights to duties instead of giving them a primary role in morality. As discourse about rights becomes derivative, it loses much of its rhetorical punch. If my right to medical care depends on your duty to provide it, my right is no longer primary, fundamental, and independent. The theory of rights then takes on all the difficulties of duty theories, especially their problems in coming to grips with individual cases. Talking about rights at first seems to promise some definite answers. If rights are derived from duties or if we need to rank them in order of importance, however, we will find rights just as vague and conflicted as duties. The right to life, for example, may be construed as the duty to care for the lives of others. As such, it becomes subject to the same questions of circumstance and degree that weakened the theory of moral duties.

The third element of a theory is its *list* of rights. The U.S. Declaration does not claim to list all rights but only certain among them. The thinking of the Supreme Court in defining a constitutional right to privacy is a good example of how complex rights arguments can become. In a famous case striking down a Connecticut law that forbade the sale of contraceptives in the state (*Griswold* v. *Connecticut*), the Supreme Court found a right to privacy in the "penumbra," literally the shadows, of the Fourteenth Amendment.

The list of rights asserted in medical situations, like the duties of health care providers, has been shifting and difficult to define. Some have held that there is a right to die or a right to die with dignity. There are also controversial claims about the right to medical care. For example, who would have the duty to provide the medical care demanded by those exercising the right?

Some of the conflicts about rights can be resolved by making a distinction between *claim rights* and *liberties,* a distinction very similar to that between positive and negative duties. Claim rights give people claims on others, while liberties guarantee the freedom of people to act as they please. The right to vote, for example, is a claim right because the citizen who is entitled to vote has a claim against election judges and polling place workers to make voting possible. Welfare rights are also claim rights, since the government has granted poor people the right to claim certain benefits. Most of the rights guaranteed in the basic documents of the United States, however, are liberties. Free speech, for example, is the right not to be interfered with in the expression of one's opinion, but it does not commit the government or anyone else to providing newspaper space or another forum for the expression of opinion.

Whether the rights under discussion are liberties or claim rights is often unclear in a medical context. People sometimes take the *right to die* to mean the right to refuse medical treatment, an assertion of the liberty to be left alone. Others believe that the right to die means that patients in certain circumstances have the right to medical help in easing their death or committing suicide. Sometimes the right to medical care means no more than that medical care should be provided without discrimination with regard to religion, race, sex, or national origin. Others argue that there is a positive or claim right to a certain level of medical care. They argue that everyone has a right to medical attention and a claim against society to obtain it.

The rights of the handicapped are typical of the complexity of the issue. Some advocates for the handicapped argue that the rights of the handicapped are liberties that may or may not be exercised. They take the right to treatment to be a liberty that one could exercise or not as one judged best, similar, perhaps, to freedom of speech. Some right to life groups, on the other hand, argue that the handicapped have claims against society to insure their life is protected. They claim that handicapped newborns, for example, have positive rights to treatment such that not treating violates their rights.

Another area of controversy with regard to claim rights is the medicaid funding of abortions. Some argue that the commitments of the federal and state governments to provide medical care for the poor, and to treat pregnancy no differently from other conditions, creates a situation in which poor women have a claim to public funding for their abortions. The other side argues that the U.S. Supreme Court's abortion decision created a liberty, a zone of privacy from government interference, but no claim to public support. They claim that public support of abortion is as optional to legislators as public support of any other project.

Conflicting claims to positive rights and our traditions of political liberty move us toward recognizing individual choices. The respect principle, which calls for us to honor the autonomy or decision-making independence of others, here coincides with those political traditions that emphasize independence. Within generous boundaries, individuals have the right to make their own choices. Once the issues in medical care cannot be resolved on the substantive ground of duty or positive rights, they become matters of the liberty of certain people to decide.

In some instances, the right to treatment is so strong a claim that denying the right is morally unacceptable. Newborns with severe but easily remedied problems, for example, have a right to treatment even though their parents, perhaps for religious reasons, do not wish to exercise that right or a hospital, facing an unpaid bill, does not wish to provide it. The children's rights, in these cases, compel treatment even over some legitimate objection.

In a far larger number of cases, however, the right to treatment is less than compelling. In these cases the question shifts from what rights require to the right to decide. Instead of asking what we should do, we ask who should decide. In terms of the moral issues that arise in medicine, should patients, relatives, physicians, or society say what should be done? The discussion of who should decide arises from the theory of moral rights and has become so important in medical ethics that it needs developed treatment.

Who Should Decide

The Patient

Patients, of course, should decide about their own medical care. As the title of the play put it: "Whose life is it anyway?" There is a very broad consensus on this point that accords with the moral theories we have already discussed. Many theories of rights hold that a person has a right to decide about his or her own medical care. Even if a person makes odd or strange decisions, the individual nonetheless has the right to make them. Moreover, physicians and nurses have a duty to help people make their own decisions, to respect their autonomous decisions, and to help carry them out. Furthermore, there are utilitarian grounds for autonomous decisions, since they are likely to produce the greatest happiness for the people most involved.

Both morality and the law recognize the right of individuals to make decisions about their own care. Patients have both a constitutional and common law right to physical integrity. As the courts declared in the landmark case of *Union Pacific Railway Co.* v. *Botsford* (1891):

No right is held more sacred, or is more carefully guarded by the common law, than the right of every individual to the possession and control of his own person, free from all restraint or interference from others, unless by clear and unquestionable authority of law. As well said by Judge Cooley, "The right to one's person may be said to be a right of complete immunity: to be let alone."

A difficulty can arise when patients ask for something that violates the moral standards of their caregivers. In a famous recent incident, a woman severely afflicted with cerebral palsy entered the psychiatric unit of a hospital because she was suicidal, but she quickly decided that she no longer wanted to be fed through a nasogastric tube and that she wanted painkillers and other medical interventions to ease her death. The hospital, the physicians, and the nurses complained that such care would compromise their morality and autonomy. In an initial finding, courts upheld the rights of health care providers to their own standards of morality and ordered the woman fed until she could be discharged from the hospital.

The same solution might be found if active euthanasia were to become legally acceptable. Since that would violate the moral standards of many in our society, only patients and health caregivers who found the practice morally acceptable would participate in it, much the way abortion is handled today.

There is a consensus that the health care decisions of conscious, rational adults are private matters. As long as they do not press their views or their care on others, society is content to leave people alone. Such cases, however, are not very common. The interesting and much more usual cases concern the care of patients who, to some degree, lack consciousness, competence, or adulthood. People who are ill are almost always compromised in one or more of these dimensions. Illness involves some loss of control. When patients are unable to decide for themselves, who is to make decisions for them?

The Kin

When patients are incapable of deciding, someone must do so for them. In the case of children, the parents usually decide. In the case of the retarded, the mentally ill, or the comatose, either a relative or a court-appointed guardian makes decisions. In many cases the situation becomes very confused because neither law nor custom makes it clear who the relevant kin are.

More important, however, is recognizing that there are two fundamentally different bases for making these decisions. The first sort of decision is a representative or *proxy* decision in which someone simply states or announces the incapacitated patient's own previously made decision about care. The second sort of decision is more difficult because it involves a *substituted* decision. Because infants, young children, and the retarded have never made any decision about their own medical care, decisions must be made for them.

The case of Edgar Jones presents a problem of proxy decision making. Edgar's past statements make it clear that he would want to be taken off the respirator, certainly after the prognosis is settled and he is plainly irreversibly comatose. His statements are not, however, documented and, although the situation may be morally clear to those involved, courts have often been reluctant to allow actions based on unverified decisions of comatose patients.

The *living will* has been introduced to enable people to express their own decisions even when they are physically unable to do so. Presently, living will legislation has been passed in more than thirty states. While the intent of the legislation is clear, there are many practical difficulties in making these laws work. Would the initial decision about resuscitating Maggie O'Sullivan be changed if she had executed a living will? The problem in that case is primarily whether her wish not to be resuscitated applies in the very unusual circumstances of her cardiac arrest. In more ordinary circumstances, her wishes are clear enough and would almost certainly be honored. Ironically, living will legislation can make it more difficult for physicians or family to carry out the wishes of patients who have neglected, as most people do, to comply with the very specific legal requirements that surround living wills. When a patient who had an opportunity to request that care be limited fails to do so, physicians may be reluctant to scale back on the level of care.

There are many interesting problems involved in knowing and carrying through on a patient's decisions, but much more difficult problems arise in the case of infants, young children, and the retarded, who have never been able to make, much less communicate, decisions of their own. Traditional morality grants parents or kin the right to make decisions for such patients. Much contemporary ethical theory, with its emphasis on autonomy, has difficulty justifying or rationalizing this tradition. One justification for the power of parents to make decisions for their children is that they are most likely to know and act in their own child's best interest. Young children should eat their vegetables, drink their milk, and stay away from candy because parents know what is good. When children grow up and learn for themselves, however, they will be happier for making their own decisions. Although this justification is usually valid, superior knowledge cannot justify parental decision making in the case of seriously

163

afflicted children. Even very bright and well-educated parents do not have the knowledge required to make decisions about the medical treatment of their child in an intensive care nursery.

The obvious reply to this suggestion is that the technical, medical knowledge that physicians and nurses have is not the human or moral knowledge needed to make good decisions for these children. We need to know what kind of life is worth living or how handicapped people are to be treated, not just how to deal with hydrocephalus or other complications of premature birth. Even granting that technical knowledge is not the issue, however, we still have not shown that even parents have the moral knowledge required. In what school do parents learn to answer these questions for their children? Physicians and nurses are not moral experts; are parents?

Two ways of thinking about substituted judgment have been proposed, both based on methods of legal decision making. The first is the "reasonable man" standard. Courts sometimes find it useful to ask what a reasonable person would do in such a situation. If someone can be shown to have acted as a reasonable person would have acted, the court may recognize the action as justifiable. The problem with this standard is that we are using it to invent the actions of infants or the retarded. Because we have no idea what a reasonable infant would do, it does not seem helpful to ask what a reasonable person would do in the infant's circumstances. Nor can the decision be judged by a "reasonable parent" standard because appropriate treatment of children with severe problems is so controversial that there are no clear models of reasonable parenting on which to base a judgment.

A similar problem arises when we try to act in the best interest of those incompetent to act on their own behalf. The expression "best interest" is borrowed from the realm of trust accounts and financial management, where trustees or guardians act in the financial interest of others. In a financial context the meaning of best interest is clear because, when it comes to money, more is better. There is no such simple standard, however, when it comes to the issues we are discussing. Is prolonged life a benefit for a handicapped infant or a demented adult, especially if that life must be lived in great pain or with little chance of independence or satisfaction? Is it ever in one's best interest to be dead? These are honest questions. Some competent adults who can make their own decisions choose to live with great pain and suffering. They live in ways many of us could never endure. Others, equally "rational" in ordinary terms, choose death. When it comes to life and other basic values involved in the medical situations discussed in this book, there is no single best interest standard to apply.

Perhaps parents are the right ones to make these decisions for their children, not because they have some special knowledge, but because they are the ones most concerned and involved with their children's care. In contrast to the previous argument, which is based on knowledge of what makes a good life, this argument is based on the duty of parents to their children and the rights of the children that correspond to these duties. Once again we can grant that assumption in usual cases, but some of the unusual cases that arise in medical ethics challenge it. Not all parents are models of care and concern for their children. Parents who are suddenly faced with caring for a handicapped child or relatives responsible for a severely damaged adult are immersed in a terrible conflict, even what might be termed a "conflict of interest." They may want to do the right thing for the patient, but they also want to do what is best for themselves and perhaps for other members of the family. There is a tragic conflict here and, without trying to assign any blame, we cannot automatically assume that parents or relatives are acting out of wholehearted concern for the patient. The relation between knowledge and concern seems to be circular. We cannot know whether, for example, parents are adequately concerned for their child if we do not know what they should do, yet only because we do not know what to do have we tuned to parental concern as our standard of judgment. If the substituted judgment of parents is difficult to justify, the cases of husbands, wives, and other relatives is even harder. Do spouses have a moral duty to tear their lives completely apart to care for one another? How far do such duties go, and how do they interact with other duties someone might have? When there is no spouse, how does one decide among the wishes, concerns, and conflicts of children and other relatives?

Providing an ethical justification for the right of kin to make decisions for one another is difficult both in theory and in practice. Suppose spouses have been at odds in recent months, even thinking seriously about divorce? Suppose, as happens often enough, that the adult children argue fiercely about the kind and amount of medical care that is appropriate for a critically ill parent; who are the relevant kin to make decisions in such situations?

The inability of relatives to make decisions is sometimes in conflict with the medical necessity that decisions be made. In such situations, physicians or nurses frequently become involved in decision making.

Doctors and Nurses

Robert Veatch of the Hastings Institute has introduced the phrase *"generalization of expertise"* to characterize the tendency of physicians to move from what he terms their legitimate area of medical expertise to assume the status of moral experts. He speaks of physicians acting as a kind of priesthood when they make decisions for others. The view that physicians and nurses should stay within their medical and technical expertise and not venture into the sphere of moral decision making is widely held in the medical ethics community. Philosophers are very wary of *paternalism* or interfering with someone's choices for that person's own good.

Physicians and nurses, however, are often drawn into making decisions for patients. Sometimes they act because the patient is unable to function autonomously and there is no cohesive or responsible family to act for the patient. On other occasions nurses and physicians influence decisions because they have a better knowledge of the patient's needs or interests than the patient. Because they know other patients and the general course of a given disease, they are often in a better position than the patients to make judgments. While not all of these examples are strictly paternalistic, they are examples of the way nurses and physicians move beyond the narrowly medical and become deeply involved in moral and human decisions.

Physicians or nurses are often involved in decisions by the way they present information or bring up questions. There is a good chance that the way information is conveyed, the values and the biases that inevitably accompany any presentation, will have a powerful impact on the decision. In the case of Christie, for example, the physician's first and most important decision is how the medical information should be presented to her father. Even the "neutral" presentation in this case is not very neutral; it contains all sorts of biases about decision making and the outcome for handicapped children.

Nurses may feel that we have exaggerated their role, but they are often closer than physicians to patients and family, especially in critical care situations when the physicians involved are not the family doctors. Physicians will often ask nurses to find out what the family wants or even to guide family discussions so that necessary decisions can be made. Neither physicians nor nurses are morally neutral, and it is difficult to see how they could be or whether they should be.

In less technically sophisticated and more stable times, the health care professional was usually the family doctor working in the community hospital. He usually knew the patient and the family, often sharing their background and values. In these circumstances it was far easier for the physician to arrive at decisions that were congruent with those of patient and family. Now it is more commonly the case that physicians and nurses are taking care of strangers. Health care providers must therefore be sensitive to the diversity of their patients' values and be reluctant to impose their own values on them.

Many philosophers, as part of their critique of paternalism, argue that physicians lack the moral standing to be involved in the moral aspects of decision making, but the tradition of physicians, the law, and the general view of society expects them to be. The Hippocratic oath demands that physicians act for the benefit of their patients and, implicitly, to determine what that benefit is. As an aspect of licensing physicians and restricting drugs, the law makes physicians the exclusive gatekeepers to certain therapies. It also requires physicians to report cases of suspected child neglect or abuse as well as certain communicable diseases. Most people in society still expect their physicians to provide personal or moral guidance. None of these functions is simply technical; their gatekeeping role inevitably involves physicians in the moral lives of their patients. If a physician believes a patient is making a mistake about his or her medical care, that physician must try to persuade the patient of the error. Ultimately, the physician may acquiesce to the patient's decision, if that is possible, resign from the case, or seek legal intervention to order treatment. The role of physicians, as defined by themselves, the law, and society, demands that they not participate in what they regard as immoral decisions.

Therefore, developing technology is not alone in generating the conflicts of medical ethics. Many of these issues arise because there is no longer a broad social consensus about the meaning of life, death, sickness, and medical care. When society confronts such problems with its own pluralism, it commonly turns to government, particularly the courts, to sort them out.

The Courts

Although the courts are only one branch of American government, they have been the one most deeply involved with the controversies in medical ethics. When the legislature becomes involved, as in Medicaid funding of abortion or the 1984 Amendments to the Child Abuse Act, the courts have been called on to review the law and its application. When the executive has acted, as in the Baby Doe regulations, the action has been quickly challenged in the courts. The courts, for better or worse, have been the main forum in which our society has usually argued the issues of medical ethics.

The fact that an issue is brought to the courts introduces a bias to the argument. Courts are more attuned to issues of individual rights than to public policy or social welfare. They worry less about what makes people

167

happy than about whether people's rights are respected. In decisions concerning the care of Karen Quinlan, Joseph Saikewicz, Brother Fox, and Claire Conroy, courts have wrestled with the issue of who has the right to decide and the limits within which court-appointed guardians may act. Some opinions have called for the courts themselves to be involved in individual cases; others have called for hospitals or nursing homes to set up procedures for making decisions within boundaries established by the courts.

In preparing their decisions, judges have consulted the writings of philosophers and theologians. As a body of significant decisions has developed, they have consulted with each other. Some recent court decisions provide exhaustive surveys of both the legal and ethical literature on decision making for comatose or extremely handicapped individuals. These decisions, as well as the latest version of the Baby Doe regulations, move in the direction of recognizing the validity of decision-making procedures other than the courts. Judges are anxious not to get involved in every difficult case that comes along. At the same time, the courts have introduced both substantive and procedural guides within which families, physicians, and health care facilities can act.

In the case of Claire Conroy, for example, the New Jersey Supreme Court wrote an eighty-three page decision spelling out the substantive and procedural rules that we quote in the Edgar Jones case. For example, it required that the ombudsman who works with nursing home patients in that state review the cases of patients for whom withdrawal of food and water is contemplated. The latest version of the Baby Doe regulations is similar in that, after setting standards of child neglect (which we quote in the cases of Christie and the Castelli baby), they recommend that hospitals establish ethics committees to apply the standards and review cases of suspected neglect. Courts are inclined to see issues in terms of rights and to resolve problems by setting up procedures. That is only natural, since courts are themselves systems of procedures to resolve conflict. Courts have also recognized that the procedures that they use are not necessarily best for resolving medical and moral issues. The *advocacy* system, which pits one side against another in hopes that conflict will bring out the truth and result in a fair settlement, does not fit medical situations well. In our cases everyone—family, nurses, physicians, hospitals—is a *patient advocate*. The problem is that they are often advocating conflicting courses of action. Moreover, bringing a case to public court involves abandoning much of the privacy to which patients and families are normally entitled. Finally, courts are resigned to settle conflict that can be settled nowhere else, and most courts believe that the issues of medical ethics can be settled by the patients, families, nurses, physicians, and hospitals most directly involved.

This discussion of the courts and how they have dealt with the issues provides an important clue to constructive moral thinking. Good moral thinking depends on something akin to procedure. The mark of good decisions, we will argue in the next chapter, is how the decisions are made.

Conclusion

We hope the conflicts among the theories that we have explained and that you find in the suggested readings do not leave you with a sense of frustration and failure. We agree that none of the theories presented provides a complete guide to good action, but we do not accept the pessimistic view that all arguments about morality are therefore futile. There is much to be learned from each of the theories discussed in this chapter, even if none is sufficient by itself. In the next chapter we will try to show how the moral theories we have been discussing can be fit together. The theory we present is not as decisive as any of the theories we have discussed, but there are important reasons why that is so.

The theory we develop flows naturally from the way in which courts arrive at their decisions. The mark of good decision making in the courts is a good process of decision making. That is the gist of our theory: that good decisions are justified by *how* they are made. The moral value of decisions depends not on what is decided or on who decides so much as on how the decision is made.

Suggestions for Further Reading

There is much more to be said about the moral problems that arise in medicine and about the philosophical theories that deal with them. We hope the preceding pages have given you an appetite for more. Here are some accessible sources for further reading in medical ethics.

There are many anthologies that include articles in philosophy and in specific issues in medical ethics. Four of the most widely available and complete are: Arras and Hunt, *Ethical Issues in Modern Medicine* (Palo Alto, Calif., 1983); Beauchamp and Walters, *Contemporary Issues in Bioethics* (Belmont, Calif., 1982); Gorovitz, Macklin, Jameton, O'Connor, and Sherwin, *Moral Problems in Medicine* (Englewood Cliffs, N.J., 1983); and Mappes and Zembaty, *Biomedical Ethics* (New York, 1986).

In addition to further readings, each of these volumes provides useful references to still more of the work in the field.

Thomas Olshewsky has written a very helpful introduction to philosophical ethics entitled *Foundations of Moral Decisions: A Dialogue* (Belmont, Calif., 1985), the final chapter of which provides an excellent bibliography. There are several contemporary treatments of ethical theory that repay the reader's serious attention, among them: John Rawls, *A Theory of Justice* (Cambridge, Mass., 1971); Smart and Williams, *Utilitarianism: For and Against* (Cambridge, Mass., 1973); and Alan Donagan, *The Theory of Morality* (Chicago, 1977). And the classics, available in numerous editions, always reward the reader: Aristotle, *Nicomachean Ethics;* Immanuel Kant, *Foundations of the Metaphysics of Morals;* and John Stuart Mill, *Utilitarianism.*

The President's Commission for the Study of Ethical Problems in Medicine and Biomedical and Behavioral Research prepared a number of outstanding volumes on specific issues in bioethics, including *Defining Death, Deciding to Forego Life-Sustaining Treatment,* and *Splicing Life.* They are published by the U.S. Government Printing Office, Washington, D.C. Current issues in medical ethics are discussed in the *Hastings Center Report,* a bimonthly publication of the Institute of Society, Ethics, and the Life Sciences. There are also a number of fine books that provide a unified view of the problems of medical ethics and that tie together much of the apparent diversity. Among them are Samuel Gorovitz, *Doctors' Dilemmas* (New York, 1982); Jonsen, Sigler, and Winslade, *Clinical Ethics* (New York, 1982); Beauchamp and Childress, *Principles of Biomedical Ethics* (New York, 1983); and Paul Ramsey, *The Patient As Person* (New Haven, Conn., 1970).

Finally, there are several works that approach the issues of medical ethics from one of the major religious traditions. Ramsey and McCormick's *Doing Evil to Achieve Good: Moral Choice in Conflict Situations* provides a dialogue between Protestantism and one side of the Roman Catholic position, while the other side of the Catholic tradition is found in Grisez and Boyle, *Life and Death with Liberty and Justice* (Notre Dame, Ind., 1979). The Jewish tradition is presented in Rosner and Bleich, *Jewish Bioethics* (New York, 1979).

Chapter 15

A Process Approach to Moral Decision Making

Most medical decisions need little ethical discussion. The child with a presumed inflamed appendix needs an operation. Although 40 percent of the appendices removed will be normal, this is accepted as the false negative rate necessary, with imperfect medical diagnostic techniques, to avoid the complications associated with waiting to be more certain. There is no ethical debate associated with the decision to operate.

When an adult has Guillain-Barre disease, a progressive inflammation of the nerves leading to increasing weakness and sometimes to insufficient respiration, there is no ethical debate about putting that individual on a respirator. Most such patients will recover and return to normal lives. The respirator is a transient part of the medical technology required to allow recovery.

For these and most other medical decisions, there is a professional and social consensus on what should be done and a relatively simple process for determining it. Benefits and costs are usually clear, duties are apparent, and the patient readily consents to the physician's proposal.

It is primarily with tough decisions—when costs are not clear and duties not obvious or when the patient's desires are different from those of the medical team—that alternative decisions may be made because the standard solutions are no longer appropriate. In such circumstances, when people do not know what should be done and it is not clear who should decide, we have found it helpful to think about how a good decision can be made, to think about the process rather than the product.

Decisions in medicine are not like those of an appellate court that has the leisure to look back over the way in which a completed case was handled. Medical decision making is prospective, looking toward a future that is necessarily uncertain and risky. As several of our cases illustrate, we must sometimes live with bad results. Living with bad outcomes is possible if we have made the decisions that led to those results in an upright and honorable way.

Conflict and tragedy raise medical and moral issues, but so do social and technological change. Medicine and morality are not fixed in stone nor do they operate in an historical vacuum. The standards of good medicine develop as new technology is introduced and as social values change. Ethics, our systematic thinking about morality, also changes with the time, culture, and circumstance. Ethical debate changes morality because new practices require new justification or criticism. Similarly, morality—what we do—may change ethics—how we think about what we do. Practice may at times lead theory, just as at other times theory may guide practice. Thus ethics, morality, and medicine have a dynamic interaction.

This interaction can be seen in some of the changes that have occurred in medical practice in recent decades. Each of the following four events introduced, or is introducing, important changes in how medicine is practiced and in how we think about those practices. In discussing these landmarks, we will begin to explain how our approach to good decision making works.

Four Medical and Moral Landmarks

The Nuremberg Trials—Informed Consent

At the end of World War II, these trials brought to light the atrocities committed by Nazi Germany against Jews, Gypsies, and other non-Aryan people. Some of these atrocities involved drafting unwilling subjects into medical experiments. As part of the legal process of prosecuting Nazis for these crimes, the tribunal at Nuremberg enunciated principles against involuntary subjection to medical experiments.

> The voluntary consent of the human subject is essential. This means that the person involved should have legal capacity to give consent; should be so situated as to be able to exercise free power of choice, without the intervention of force, fraud, deceit, duress, overreaching or other ulterior form of constraint or coercion; and should have sufficient knowledge and comprehension of the subject matter in-

volved as to enable him to make an understanding and enlightened decision.

Trials of War Criminals before the Nuremberg Military Tribunals, Washington, D.C., U.S. Government Printing Office, 1948

Examination of the Nazi crimes gradually altered our thinking not only about consent from human subjects in medical experiments, but also about everyday therapeutic procedures. What was implicit in medical practice for centuries was brought to the surface by these historic trials.

Response to the revelations at Nuremberg was not instantaneous. Even after the declaration of Helsinki (a statement of the Eighteenth World Medical Assembly meeting in Helsinki, Finland in 1964), which reaffirmed the moral rejection of experiments without adequate consent, many researchers did not see the connection between their work and the Nazi medical experiments. The U.S. Public Health Service, for example, continued its observation of untreated syphilis until news reporters broke the story in 1972, over 25 years after it was discovered that penicillin effectively and easily treated the disease.

It was even more difficult for many in the medical community to connect the notion of informed consent with therapy. Many thought that by virtue of presenting themselves for examination, patients implicitly gave doctors both a request for a diagnosis and an authorization of treatment. They viewed truly informed consent as an ideal beyond the grasp of ordinary medical practice. Asking for consent after explaining all of the risks of complications and side effects seemed both excessively time consuming and potentially frightening to the patients.

Several of the cases in this book illustrate how difficult it is to inform patients or relatives of all the medical facts that are important in making good decisions. For example, Maggie (Chapter 1) does not want to be put "on those damn machines." Does she mean she does not want to be resuscitated after a brief, medication-induced cardiac arrest? Can you obtain informed consent in advance for all possible contingencies? When you seek informed consent from Christie's parents (Chapter 9), you have to inform them of the probable outcome. What bias do you use when you provide the information? What happens if parental refusal is intolerable? While you need Rosa's permission to discontinue treatment of Tom (Chapter 5), would you consider letting her see the discomfort caused by his treatment as a way of shaping her decision or would that be a form of coercion?

There is consensus that informed consent is a requirement for morally responsible medicine, but there remains an ongoing discussion of how understandable information can and should be given and geunine consent obtained. The moral value of informed consent depends on the process of carrying this out.

Ironically, informed consent has generated problems in its own turn. What should be done when patients, or relatives acting for them, refuse consent to procedures that the medical community or society at large deems beneficial?

The Johns Hopkins Baby

In the early 1970s this case provoked a thorough reconsideration of the treatment of newborns with major handicaps. A baby was born at the Johns Hopkins Hospital with Down's syndrome and duodenal atresia, a blockage of the upper part of the intestine. Without surgery to open the obstruction, it would have been impossible to feed the baby. After lengthy consultation with senior physicians at the hospital who recommended the operation, the baby's parents decided not to consent to the proposed operation. The infant was placed in a back room on the ward, and during the following week the baby died of starvation and dehydration.

At that time such decisions were not rare. There was no established view in the medical community, and there had been little public debate on the issue. A standard recommendation for many otherwise healthy Down's syndrome infants was that they be institutionalized immediately so that the parents would not become too attached to them. A life spent in an institution was the common fate of such children. Community services and support for the retarded were minimal. Surgical treatment of mentally impaired babies was considered optional because little medical, educational, or social support was available for them even after "successful" medical treatment. Vigorous treatment was therefore not considered a benefit to the children, much less to their families or society.

Thinking about care of the retarded was beginning to change, however. After considerable reflection and discussion, Dr. Robert Cooke, chairman of the Department of Pediatrics at Johns Hopkins, and officials from the Kennedy Foundation decided to recreate the drama of the decision in a film that was used as a starting point for a panel discussion on the ethics of treating children with Down's syndrome. Challenging the assumptions underlying the original decision, members of the panel suggested new ways to help parents cope with their Down's children and encouraged the development of community support services. They criticized the practice of institutionalizing the retarded. They also challenged the exclusive right of the parents to decide, arguing that either foster care or adoption were practical alternatives when parents were unable to cope with a handicapped child.

The political prominence of the Kennedy family and their commitment to helping the retarded also fostered social change. A new law passed in 1974, the Educational Rights of the Handicapped Act, ultimately entitled each handicapped child to an individualized treatment plan in a public educational facility. Facilities for community living and work, although still inadequate, are gradually replacing institutions for the retarded.

For a number of years after the publicity surrounding the "Hopkins baby," when an infant with Down's syndrome required surgery, discussions about the child's rights, the benefits of surgery or other treatment, and a multitude of moral considerations were held among the parents, physicians, and others involved in the case. A consensus gradually evolved. This common view of the prognosis and appropriate care of the retarded is now so strong that, when a Down's syndrome child is born with an associated problem, the presentation to the parents consists mainly of explaining the need for and benefit of corrective procedures. Medicine informs and parents consent. The decision-making process no longer deals with all the ambiguity of individual decisions. (We agree with the President's Commission on Biomedical Ethics and the vast majority of commentators in medical ethics that the much publicized Baby Doe case in Bloomington, Indiana, was an unusual and unjustifiable exception to this consensus.) Not operating has become an intolerable choice.

With all the benefits of hindsight, it is clear that the original decision at Johns Hopkins was morally unacceptable. What has changed? In the case of Down's syndrome, the medical facts are the same, but social attitudes and support have changed dramatically. Our moral sensitivity toward the handicapped has become more acute, and we have become more willing to nurture and support them. As our moral view of the handicapped has changed, so have the boundaries of what is acceptable. Changes in morality have led to changes in medical practice.

Spina Bifida, Technology, and the Nonretarded Handicapped Infant

The attention initially focused on newborns with Down's syndrome gradually spread to other handicapped infants, those with physical defects but no intellectual impairment. Children with spina bifida pose different questions about quality of life for the handicapped (see Chapter 9). In the 1950s few children with spina bifida were treated. The great risks of operating on the newborn and technical problems with shunts for hydrocephalus were major deterrents to intervention. The prevailing view at the time was that medical care should be given only to those who survived

175

to 1 year of age and who then showed promise of good mental function.

Technical advances in perinatal surgery and anesthesia and in shunts to drain excess fluid from the brain improved the prospects of early intervention. In the late 1950s and early 1960s a group in Sheffield, England, showed that early surgery dramatically increased the survival of a newborn with spina bifida. Euthusiasm for aggressive treatment quickly spread, and most infants with spina bifida were treated. In contrast to the situation with Down's syndrome, technology led to the change in treatment of spina bifida.

In 1971 Dr. John Lorber, one of the leaders of the Sheffield group, reviewed his experience with the children he had treated and concluded that since half the children given vigorous therapy died anyway and a substantial portion of the survivors were severely impaired, perhaps not all such infants should be treated. He suggested *selection* at birth to reduce the resources committed to both those who would die anyway and those who would survive with substantial impairments. Lorber published a series of articles (e.g., Results of treatment of Myelomeningocele. *Developmental Medicine and Child Neurology* 14:304, 1972), proposing criteria based on medical indications for selecting those who should *not* be treated.

The proposed change from virtually obligatory treatment to selection was also widely, but not universally, adopted. Whereas the shift from no treatment to aggressive treatment has caused no ethical debate, the notion of selection raised the issue: "Now we can do it, but should we?" Lorber's position stimulated a vigorous debate about the treatment of nonretarded handicapped children and their quality of life.

After a decade this debate has led to the consensus that we should treat most infants with spina bifida. Almost all children who will ultimately walk with or without braces are treated at birth. Most children who will require massive bracing or wheelchairs are also treated. It is only in this latter category that significant dialogue with parents about consent for treatment still occurs.*

There is now controversy over the use and limits of technology for treating very small premature newborns. Depending on the size of the infant (birthweight 1 to 3 pounds) and the gestational age, the survival rate of these premature infants may vary from 10 to 70 percent, and the outcome may vary from normal to profoundly retarded with severe cerebral palsy. However, unlike the situation of the child with Down's syn-

---

* It is of interest to note that with new techniques for diagnosing such problems as Down's syndrome and spina bifida in utero, there is increasing social and legal pressure to test all women and to abort affected fetuses. The ethics of this paradox—treating all survivors and aborting detected fetuses—deserves further exploration.

drome or spina bifida, there is rarely one big decision to be made, but rather a series of smaller decisions. The outcome of each of these smaller decisions is unpredictable, and their effects may be cumulative, thus the phrase "nibbling away in the nursery."

Our recognition of the quality of life of retarded and physically handicapped individuals has improved, but we are also more conscious of the cost of their care. We recognize their rights as persons, although our concept of "person" is more complex and clouded. While we are still anxious to respect parental autonomy, decisions not to treat all but the most seriously compromised newborns are no longer made solely by individual parents or physicians, but increasingly involve an independent ethics committee and society as a whole.

The debate in the U.S. about these issues has recently focused on the Baby Doe regulations. While the latest version of these regulations (published in the *Federal Register,* April 15, 1985, 45 CFR, Part 1340, pp. 14878–901, and cited in Chapters 9 and 12) is not ideal, it is a notable improvement over an earlier version that was recently struck down by the Supreme Court. The regulations currently in force developed from a remarkable consensus of liberal and conservative politicians, medical professionals and their associations, and advocates for the handicapped. They attempt to insure that infants who stand to profit from treatment are treated, that those for whom treatment would be futile or inhumane are not subjected to unwarranted therapy, and that parents and society are included in decisions. The social consensus behind these regulations evolved from the self-criticism that began with the public discussion of the baby born at Johns Hopkins.

Karen Quinlan and Claire Conroy— Technology Extending Unconscious Existence

At one time the elderly were cared for at home and typically died of pneumonia or the complications of a stroke or heart attack. Pneumonia used to be called "the old man's friend." Antibiotics ended that "friendship." At one time the individual who required respiratory support died. When tank respirators became available, they were not suitable for the elderly or for long-term use. The development of good respirators in the 1960s and 1970s has been a boon to many children and adults with acute respiratory problems. Their use has made it possible to extend many lives, some even after the ability to function consciously has been irretrievably lost. Nutrition by tube feeding (see Chapter 7) has further increased our ability to prolong life.

Karen Quinlan's was the first case to draw widespread attention to the capacity of modern medicine to sustain irreversibly comatose patients on a respirator. Claire Conroy's case can be seen as extending the question of respirator support of the comatose or severely damaged patient to that of feeding. The New Jersey Supreme Court ruled in the case of Karen Quinlan that the use of a respirator to maintain life was not always required. In Claire Conroy's case, the same court held that, under substantially more limited circumstances, even feeding is not mandatory. These cases, therefore, have moved to the center of a public debate about the level of support that should be given to irreversibly comatose patients.

Respirators are now routine in intensive care units, and the feeding of children and adults through tubes to the stomach or veins is an everyday occurrence on the wards. Access to air and nutrition would seem to be basic, but are there situations where they may be "heroic" or futile?

When we look at some of the terms of the current debate over discontinuing treatment of the elderly and comatose—living will, death with dignity, heroic measures, vegetative state—it is plain that the argument is far from closure. How can we consider quality of life without starting down the slippery slope toward killing those judged not to have very much life? How can we take the rights of incompetent patients seriously without locking ourselves into rigid programs of aggressively treating all such patients no matter what the circumstances of their lives? How can we be practical about who is to make decisions without setting up a single individual as a tyrant over others? In the following section we will sketch our approach to working out responses to such questions.

Good Decision Making

Good decisions are marked by openness to all the medical information that is available, to the patient and to all who are involved with the patient's care, whether as relatives or as professionals; and to the cultures, subcultures, and society of which the patient is a member. We think of openness as a practical instrument of moral criticism and self-criticism.

The events we have discussed show how people can close themselves off from a morally significant aspect of a medical and human situation. The Nazis ignored the humanity of their victims. Some recent instances of allowing newborns with Down's syndrome to die have come close to that. Physicians have closed themselves off from the needs of their patients or their families, as in the Quinlan case, and patients have sometimes tried to force physicians to act against their consciences. Patients, family members, physicians, and nurses sometimes try to exclude legitimately involved persons from decisions.

Good, open decisions rely on good facts or at least on the best knowledge currently available. Physicians are not omniscient, but they are responsible for obtaining the latest and most accurate medical information. Good decisions are also open both to the views of others involved in the situation and to outside opinion. In this way the decision makers are assured of multiple points of view and become aware of their own bias. This also means that varied ethical theories will enter into the decision-making process.

Good decision-making processes can come to different conclusions in essentially identical cases. This does not mean, however, that any answer will do or even that a widely based social consensus is necessarily correct. What was once widely accepted treatment of the retarded is now recognized as insufficient and morally culpable.

Tolerance is the public or political dimension of the open decision making we advocate. Differences in viewpoint and value are inherent in the complex moral and human situations confronting medical ethics. Tolerance involves being open to those differences. As our historical examples show, excluding values or legitimately interested parties from consideration leads to the narrowness of view that characterizes bad actions.

Unfortunately, tolerance too often is identified with moral relativism or lack of clarity in ethical theory. We see tolerance as a middle ground between dogmatism on the one hand and moral relativism on the other. Dogmatism can take many forms, only some of which are readily recognizable. Lucille Adams (Chapter 9) represents one form of dogmatism insofar as she might demand aggressive treatment of every newborn no matter how poor the prognosis or painful and crippling the treatment. Dr. Bernstein (Chapter 12) exhibits a similar dogmatism when he advocates using all available medical technology. But equally dogmatic are those who would give parents complete discretion in making decisions for their children. Even a predominant focus on informed consent can become a form of dogmatism. All these apparently different attitudes share the common moral failure involved in fastening on a single aspect of a complex moral situation and then proceeding to make it into a moral absolute.

There must be limits to tolerance, of course. Failure to treat a child with a mildly handicapping condition is intolerable: it ignores the child's potential for a fulfilling life. While we are more inclined to tolerate aggressive treatment than unjustifiable nontreatment, there may be no sufficient reason to tolerate futile and painful treatment of surely fatal diseases, even when patients or relatives demand that "something be done."

179

Although physicians may tolerate wide divergences in the decisions of their patients, they have an obligation to assure that both the patients and they themselves understand the risks, benefits, and consequences of a proposed course of action. Physicians also must decide whether a patient's decisions are within their own (the physicians') limits of tolerance. If a physician cannot accept a patient's decision, then he or she should withdraw from the case or refer the patient to another physician.

While tolerance is a relatively passive virtue, the active virtue of medicine is beneficence. Medicine is a helping profession, striving to produce benefits for patients. Physicians and nurses try to meet the needs of others, but an excess of beneficence may overwhelm patients and lead to paternalism. Although the beneficent actions of medical professionals have generally served both patients and society well, the power of modern medicine easily can convert beneficence to arrogance. With growing confidence in their ability to help patients, physicians sometimes help them to live or die in ways those individuals disapprove.

Both the general public and the philosophical community have complained of the arrogance of medicine. Some seem to prefer that physicians restrict themselves to purely technical matters and refrain from introducing any bias in the patient's decision making. We think this attitude pushes the pendulum too far. Decisions should be made both by patients, with the advice and consent of their caregivers, *and* by physicians, with the consent of their well-informed patients. Physicians possess enormous power to shape patients' decisions both by what they tell them and by what they do not say. Their tone of voice, their emphasis on the positive or negative, their body language, and all that is involved in human communication structure the information patients receive (see Chapter 9). At the same time, patients can withdraw from a physician's care. More subtly, patients can refuse to comply with prescribed treatment, distort their report of symtoms, or in other ways frustrate their physicians' plans. None of this leads to good medicine.

Good decisions result from an interactive, even symbiotic, relationship between physician and patient, but the relationship also includes family members, friends, nurses, and other members of the health care team. All participants in the process must work within the limits of their own tolerance. This is true both for decisions to limit treatment and for decisions to start treatment. Good processes of decision making require that all parties tolerate the diversity of others' viewpoints and work toward defining and achieving a consensus about what is best for the patient.

The classical discussion of medical ethics focused on the Hippocratic tradition and emphasized acting for the benefit of the patient. Abuses of beneficence such as the paternalism of well-intentioned but authoritarian physicians helped bring autonomy and informed consent to the fore as a counterbalance. The principle of autonomy was readily accepted because it is so closely connected with the traditions of liberty that inform political discussion in the U.S.

In rushing to insure individual liberty and autonomy, however, our culture is in some danger of pushing to an opposite extreme. We too often, it seems, ignore the fact that the principal barrier to a patient's liberty is debilitating disease. In helping to restore health, medicine often restores freedom as well. Overemphasizing the right of patients to refuse medical care can obscure the benefits of effective medicine. At this time we are less afraid of a little paternalism than we are of the social isolation and neglect of good health care that can follow from overstressing autonomy.

We are concerned that a balance be restored. Given the difficulties of conveying meaningful medical information to patients and the inevitable limits that disease imposes on freedom and autonomy, informed consent is not, by itself, adequate to insure morally good decisions. The beneficent tradition of medicine needs to be recognized as the engine that drives researchers and caregivers to help those who depend on them. It is an irreplaceable element of good morals and good medicine.